Physiology and Nutrition
for Amateur Wrestling

Physiology and Nutrition for Amateur Wrestling

Charles Paul Lambert, PhD
Relentless Human Performance, LLC
International Network of Wrestling Researchers
USA Wrestling Leader

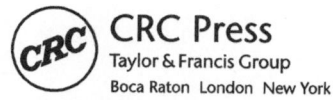

CRC Press
Taylor & Francis Group
Boca Raton London New York

CRC Press is an imprint of the
Taylor & Francis Group, an **informa** business

First edition published 2021
by CRC Press
6000 Broken Sound Parkway NW, Suite 300, Boca Raton, FL 33487-2742

and by CRC Press
2 Park Square, Milton Park, Abingdon, Oxon, OX14 4RN

Library of Congress Cataloging-in-Publication Data
Names: Lambert, Charles Paul, 1965- author.
Title: Physiology and nutrition for amateur wrestling / by Charles Paul Lambert, PhD.
Description: First edition. | Boca Raton : CRC Press, 2020. | Includes bibliographical references and index. | Summary: "Physiology and Nutrition for Amateur Wrestling is essential reading for amateur wrestlers and their coaches with a desire to learn about physiological training and nutrition for their sport. Written by Charles Lambert, PhD, a competitive wrestler and academic expert in high-intensity exercise"—Provided by publisher.
Identifiers: LCCN 2020013310 (print) | LCCN 2020013311 (ebook) | ISBN 9780367370947 (paperback) | ISBN 9780367375171 (hardback) | ISBN 9780429354779 (ebook)
Subjects: LCSH: Wrestling—Physiological aspects. | Wrestlers--Nutrition.
Classification: LCC RC1220.W73 L36 2020 (print) | LCC RC1220.W73 (ebook) | DDC 796.812—dc23
LC record available at https://lccn.loc.gov/2020013310
LC ebook record available at https://lccn.loc.gov/2020013311

ISBN: 978-0-367-37517-1 (hbk)
ISBN: 978-0-367-37094-7 (pbk)
ISBN: 978-0-429-35477-9 (ebk)

Typeset in Times
by codeMantra

Contents

PART 1   Physiological Basis for Wrestling

PART 2   *Nutrition for Amateur Wrestling*
           Fueling the Machine

Purpose

To educate high-school and college coaches and wrestlers on physiological training for amateur wrestling and nutrition for amateur wrestling.

Author

Charles Paul Lambert, PhD was born in Toledo, Ohio May 26, 1965. He was brought up in a suburb of Toledo, Sylvania, Ohio where he wrestled, played football and some baseball in junior high school and high school at Sylvania Southview High School. Noteworthy of his wrestling career was that he achieved 50 takedowns in his senior year and was awarded the Takedown Trophy. Also, in 1981, under the auspices of the Amateur Athletic Union (AAU), he was second in the State Greco-Roman Tournament, where he lost in the finals to Joe Ghezzi 0-6, being underarm spun with a go behind six times. Dr. Lambert was 19-6 in his senior year for Sylvania Southview, a three-year varsity letter winner, and a co-captain in his senior year. With regard to football, he started at varsity offensive guard (145 lbs) as a sopho-more, junior, and senior and started at inside linebacker his senior year and was the runner-up or leading tackler his senior season. He was also co-captain of the football team in his senior year.

Upon graduation from Sylvania Southview High School in 1983, Dr. Lambert entered the University of Toledo and graduated with a 3.55 Grade Point Average (GPA) in Human Performance (now Exercise Science) in 1988. This GPA, along with research experience and publications with Michael G. Flynn, PhD, helped him get a "free ride" to graduate school at the Human Performance Lab at Ball State University. Dr. Lambert excelled in this fertile academic setting, and it was the most rewarding two years of his life, achieving a 3.93 GPA (including a year of Biochemistry in the Chemistry Department) and learning a great deal about applied physiology research, including rehydration after dehydration, under Dr. David L. Costill. After graduation in 1990, Dr. Lambert worked in Dr. Ron Maughan's lab at the University of Aberdeen Medical School, Aberdeen, Scotland for one year. This also was a great experience for Dr. Lambert, studying mechanisms of fluid replace-ment and metabolism during high-intensity exercise. Dr. Lambert then worked with John O. Holloszy, MD for one year at the Washington University Medical School. Dr. Lambert completed his PhD at the University of Toledo in 1997, again under the auspices of Dr. Michael G. Flynn. His area of research for his dissertation was Exercise and Immunology. His Doctoral GPA was 3.88.

After teaching for a year at Eastern Michigan University, Dr. Lambert became a Post-Doctoral fellow in the Nutrition, Metabolism, and Exercise lab of William J. Evans, PhD, within the Department of Geriatrics at the University of Arkansas for Medical Sciences (UAMS). Dr. Lambert spent eight years primarily perform-ing research at UAMS, publishing some 21 papers in those eight years, and pro-curing two National Institutes of Health grants dealing with muscle hypertrophy in the elderly. He was an assistant professor when he left UAMS. After UAMS, Dr. Lambert went to Washington University School of Medicine for two years, bring-ing 90% of his salary with him in grant money. He was a research assistant professor in the Department of Geriatrics and Nutritional Science within Internal Medicine.

There, Dr. Lambert completed his NIH/National Institute on Aging R21 grant titled: "Effects of Albuterol on Muscle Protein Synthesis".

Dr. Lambert left Washington University and went to the University of Louisville, where he taught, performed research, and mentored students. After two years, Dr. Lambert left University of Louisville to be with his aging father. After a number of years away from academia, Dr. Lambert taught for Stautzenberger College for two years. Currently, Dr. Lambert is writing and applying for Tenure Track positions in Exercise Physiology/Science.

Dr. Lambert has published ~70 peer-reviewed papers and has been the first author on at least 30 of these. He has acquired two National Institutes of Health grants and other various grants. He is a member of the International Network of Wrestling Researchers, a Bronze Certified Coach through USA Wrestling, and was a Mat Official for USA Wrestling for four years. In his spare time, Dr. Lambert is a Powerlifter, having Bench Pressed 336.2 lbs in competition at the age of 54 which qualified him for the USPA World Championships and is currently ranked 4th in the USPA/USA in Powerlifting. Recently, Dr. Lambert qualified for the USPA Nationals with a total 1,102 lbs.

1 Introduction

Amateur Wrestling is a high-intensity intermittent activity which is both aerobic and anaerobic, lasting 6–7 minutes. As a result, a wrestler should train both aerobically and anaerobically based on Specific Adaptations to Imposed Demands (SAID Principle). The physiological components of wrestling success can be broken down into: "Maximal Power Output", "Entire Match Wrestling Power Output", and "flexibility". "Maximal Power Output" is primarily governed by maximal force output, while "Entire Match Wrestling Power Output" is dependent on Maximal Force Output, Anaerobic Capacity, and Critical Power. "Maximal Force Output" is maximal strength, "Anaerobic Capacity" is the total ability to generate energy anaerobically, and "Critical Power" is the maximal sustainable power output that is entirely aerobic. Flexibility is just a measure of joint range of motion.

The duration of an amateur wrestling match is usually 6–7 minutes long (Figure 1.1). As such, a match is performed at approximately 95%–100% of maximal oxygen consumption (VO_2max) (Gleeson, Greenhaff, and Maughan 1988; Katz et al. 1986). The duration and intensity (intermittently above 100% of VO_2max; i.e., scrambles, throws, and lifts) of a match dictate that both anaerobic and aerobic sources of energy are utilized. Thus, a wrestler should train both anaerobically and aerobically. This is because of the SAID principle. The SAID principle stands for Specific Adaptations to Imposed Demands, which means you get what you train for. If you train for strength you will achieve strength, and if you train for muscular endurance

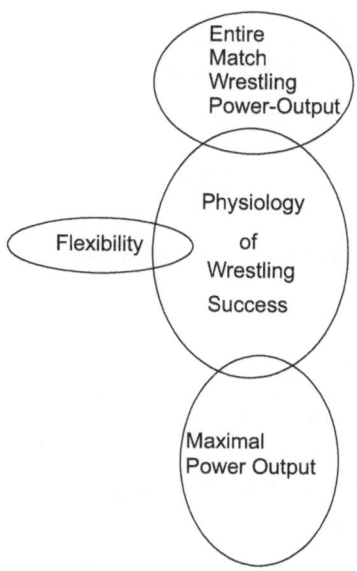

FIGURE 1.1 Physiological components of amateur wrestling success.

you will achieve muscular endurance. The philosophy behind this book is that if you want the highest possible sustained power output of 6–7 minutes, you must be able to generate very high instantaneous power outputs whenever the opportunity arises in a match or when the wrestler makes the opportunity for that very high instantaneous power output to happen. Therefore, you have to develop the function (physiology) of the body to both maintain very high sustained power outputs and develop the body to generate very high instantaneous power outputs. An additional component of wrestling success is flexibility or joint range of motion. Likewise, you have to eat (nutrition) to maintain high power outputs for 6–7 minutes (possibly many times in one day and/or multiple days) and also generate high instantaneous power outputs. In essence, you need to train and eat for both high force-generating capacity for the full 6–7 minutes (possibly multiple times a day) and to train and eat so that you can generate very high forces within 1–2 seconds. When sustained for only 30 seconds, this sustained power output is called "Anaerobic Capacity" (i.e., obtained from a Wingate 30-second cycle ergometer test). We will call this 6–7-minute sustained power output "Entire Match Wrestling Power Output" (Figure 1.2).

And clearly the instantaneous power output is called "Maximal Power Output" (Figure 1.3).

Training for these two types of Power Outputs is quite different, but the optimal nutrition for "Entire Match Wrestling Power Output" training will overlap and be more than adequate for the "Maximal Power Output" training. The great majority of

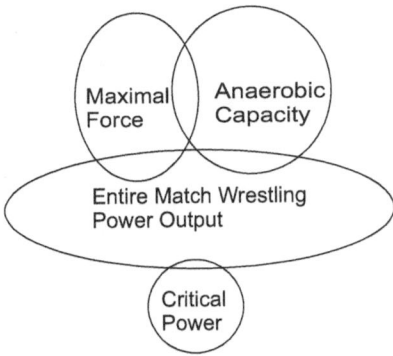

FIGURE 1.2   Components of entire match wrestling power output.

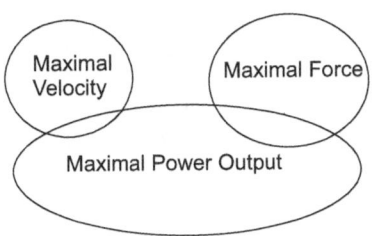

FIGURE 1.3   Components of Maximal Power Output.

this book will be dedicated to helping the wrestler and coach determine what is the best way to train and eat for "Entire Match Wrestling Power Output" and "Maximal Power Output".

KEY POINTS

1. Wrestling is fueled by both anaerobic and aerobic metabolism.
2. SAID Principle dictates the adaptions obtained from training.
3. A wrestler needs to eat and train for Maximal Power Output and Entire Match Wrestling Power Output.

2 Positive Benefits of Wrestling

EFFECTS OF WRESTLING ON PHYSICAL FITNESS

Wrestling is an activity that, for the match taken as a whole, is conducted at or just below VO_2max (Lambert and Jones 2010). As a result of specific adaptations to imposed demands, wrestling is an excellent activity for improving the maximal fitness level (VO_2max). Training for wrestling, if not the best, is a best practice for improving maximal fitness level. One of the reasons this is the case is that both the upper body and lower body are used aerobically and anaerobically, similar with cross-country skiing, but more intense (a higher percentage of VO_2max). The greater the muscle mass involvement, the greater the oxygen consumption (VO_2) and stress on the cardiovascular system, and hence the greater the adaptation. Clearly, this is a positive selling point of amateur wrestling when compared with other youth sports. Another selling point is the transfer of wrestling physiological components to other sports, such as strength and anaerobic capacity, being transferred to football and field events, aerobic fitness being transferred to soccer, track, and cross-country. Additionally, as far as skills, wrestling transfers well to football, with regard to, tackling and blocking (Table 2.1, Figure 2.1).

Wrestling (and those that have done it can attest to this) is one of the most physically demanding sports you can undertake. As such, the energy expenditure (kcals) during wrestling is quite high. Although there are no direct data I know about, data from Judo (a close relative to amateur wrestling) suggests that a Judoka expends 13.8 kcals/minute (Brooks, Fahey, and Baldwin 2005). A quick calculation yields 828 kcals/hour. Clearly, wrestling and Judo result in an extreme energy expenditure per unit time. The body composition and fitness benefits of wrestling are great because of their large energy expenditure. With this type of caloric expenditure who needs to diet? We should promote our sport as one that is great for kids because of its beneficial effect on body fat and physical fitness, without dieting. Imagine if

---

TABLE 2.1.

Physiological Benefits of Consistent *Live* Wrestling across the Life Span

Strength

Agility

Muscular endurance

Maximal aerobic fitness (VO_2max) via high-intensity interval training

Enhanced energy expenditure

Improved body composition

Improved cognitive function

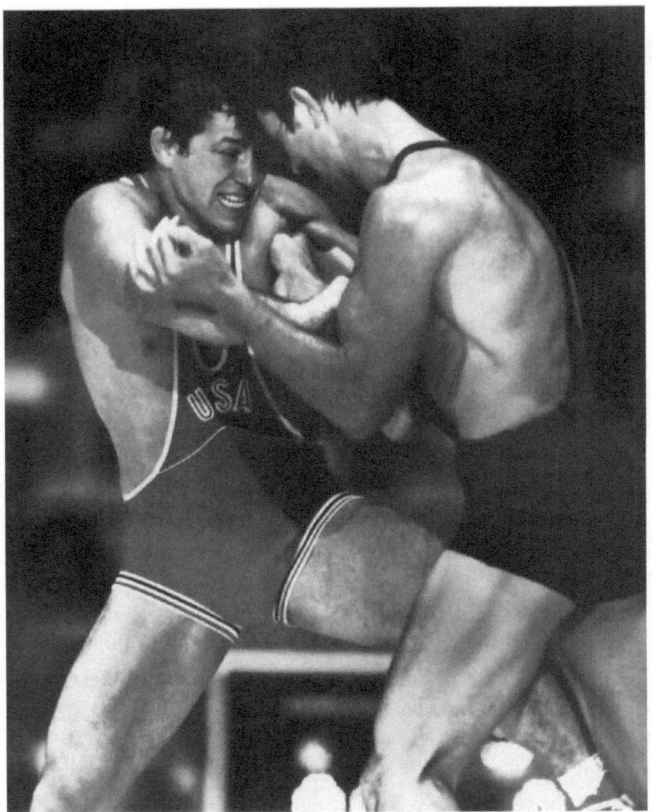

FIGURE 2.1   Steve Fraser, retouched.

every kid playing video games after school was a wrestler? The childhood obesity epidemic would be over without affecting school lunches. Couple the energy expenditure of wrestling with the fact that wrestling is a low-impact (knees and ankles) sport, compared with a sport where running is involved, and you have the perfect fitness regimen. Thus, wrestling may be the best sport for treating the childhood obesity epidemic.

EFFECTS OF PHYSICAL ACTIVITY ON COGNITIVE FUNCTION

Exercise, including wrestling, has beneficial effects on childrens' cognitive function and academic achievement. In a thorough review of the literature, the American College of Sports Medicine (Donnely et al. 2016) has taken a position stand on the effects of acute and chronic exercise on cognitive function and academic achievement in children. From this review of the literature, it is clear that physical activity has positive effects on both cognitive function and academic achievement. As a result, there is sufficient reason to keep physical education programs in schools and for keeping wrestling programs at high schools and middle schools. These reasons are for more than just the effects of these programs on physical fitness and body composition. One caveat here is that wrestling with substantial weight cutting or insufficient carbohydrate intake may actually impair cognitive function through hypoglycemia (low blood sugar). Thus, wrestling is a great activity if coupled with sound nutritional practices.

KEY POINTS

1. Wrestling is an excellent way to train for aerobic fitness.
2. Wrestling is an excellent way to optimize body composition because of the high energy (caloric output).
3. Sports in general without significant weight cutting have a highly beneficial effect on cognitive function.

Part 1

Physiological Basis for Wrestling

3 Skeletal Muscle

Skeletal muscle contraction involves many muscle proteins as well as sodium (Na^+) and potassium (K^+) and adenosine triphosphate (ATP), and vital ions such as magnesium (Mg^{2+}) and calcium (Ca^{2+}). The whole muscle contracts by way of individual sarcomere shortening. A sarcomere is Z-line to Z-line. After the ATP is broken down, the myosin head (thick filament head) cocks, and the release of Ca^{2+} from the sarcoplasmic reticulum upon electrical stimulation through the T-tubule system ensures that Ca^{2+} binds to troponin. Once the Ca^{2+} binds to troponin, tropomyosin moves away from the myosin head binding site on actin. The myosin head binds and muscle contraction ensues—myosin head moving actin. The ATP then binds to the myosin head again, is split and released from actin, Ca^{2+} is taken back up into the sarcoplasmic reticulum and relaxation ensues, or the process of shortening continues if Ca^{2+} is still in the local environment.

There are three kinds of muscle: skeletal, cardiac, and smooth. In this chapter I will discuss Skeletal Muscle. Skeletal Muscle has a striated appearance and about 100 nuclei per muscle cell. This large number of nuclei is important because it allows for a great deal of protein synthesis to go on as a result of the great deal of DNA contained within the 100 nuclei (Figure 3.1).

Skeletal Muscle is designed for contraction; or in other words shortening. The two main proteins in skeletal muscle are actin and myosin. Actin is called the thin filament while myosin is called the thick filament. The heads of the thick filament pull the thin filaments toward one another and the Z-lines become closer together (Figure 3.2). The functional unit of skeletal muscle is the sarcomere from Z-line to Z-line. When a number of sarcomeres contract the whole muscle shortens. When the whole muscle shortens, bones and their associated tissues are moved closer together called flexion or are moved farther apart called extension. Within each muscle fiber or cell are the myofibrils. The outer covering on a muscle cell or fiber is

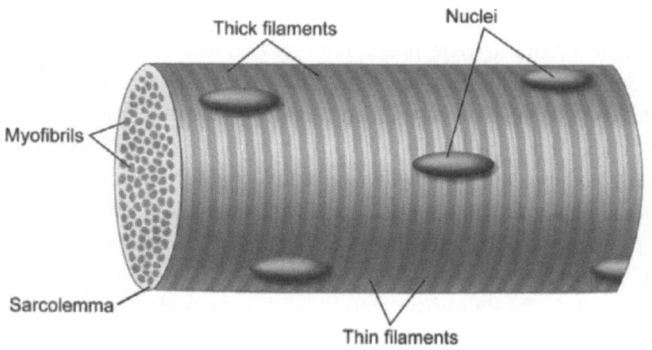

FIGURE 3.1   Skeletal muscle fiber.

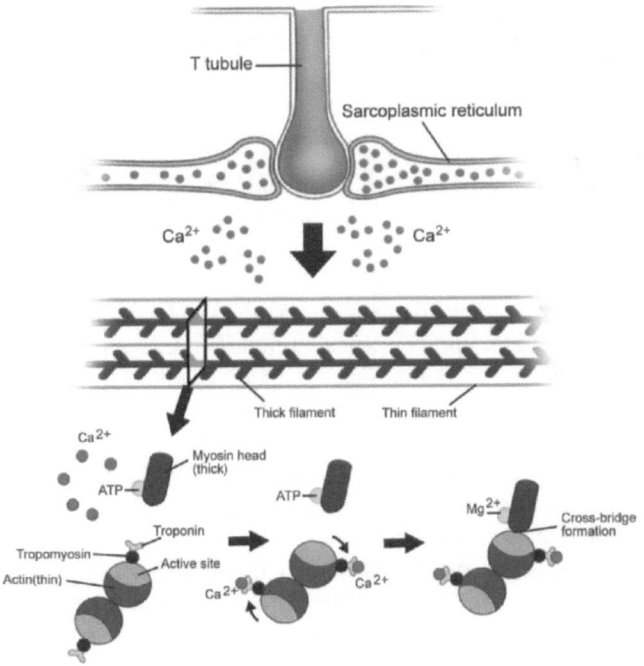

FIGURE 3.2   Muscle contraction.

called endomysium. Perimysium surrounds a bundle of muscle fibers called fasicles, while epimysium covers the whole muscle. The sarcolemma is the plasma membrane of cell membrane for a muscle cell/fiber. Once an impulse from the motor portion of the nervous system excites the sarcolemma to a point of depolarization, the impulse travels to the T-tubule system which is connected to the sarcoplasmic reticulum. The sarcoplasmic reticulum houses calcium. Excitation of the T-tubule system results in the release of Ca^{2+} by the Sarcoplasmic Reticulum. The released calcium binds to the protein troponin which is bound to tropomyosin which covers the binding sites on actin. Once the troponin binds Ca^{2+} tropomyosin moves exposing the binding sites on actin for the myosin head. The myosin head then pulls the actin closer together and the sarcomere contracts. The ATP then binds to the myosin head releasing it from actin, Ca^{2+} is taken back up into the Sarcoplasmic Reticulum and the muscle cell relaxes. The splitting of ATP by an enzyme named myosin ATPase acts to cause the myosin head to cock into the ready position getting ready to pull actin closer together. This occurs again and again during a muscle contraction in a ratchet-like fashion pulling the actin closer and closer together. This is called cross-bridge cycling (McComas 1996).

As discussed in the Metabolism section ATP is provided in one of the six ways. First, stored ATP can be used; second, Phosphocreatine (PCr) can be used to resythesize ATP via PCr+ADP $\diamond$ ATP+Cr reaction. Third, glycogenolysis (the breakdown of glycogen) and anaerobic glycolysis can be used to make small amounts of ATP with Lactic Acid production. Fourth, glycogenolysis and aerobic metabolism (Krebs Cycle and Electron Transport Chain) can be used to produce a large amount of ATP utilizing the mitochondria and oxygen. Fifth, circulating blood glucose can be used aerobically (with oxygen) to produce a similar amount of ATP as that derived from muscle-bound glycogen. Sixth, fat can be used in the presence of carbohydrate to form a very large amount of ATP, but oxygen has to be available in great quantities; meaning this likely only occurs without a drop in power output during prolonged submaximal exercise where oxygen is abundant (McCartney et al. 1986). An important concept in muscle is the energy charge of the cell which is the [ATP+ADP+AMP]. ADP is Adenosine Diphosphate and AMP is Adenosine Monophosphate. From these three substrates we can acquire high-energy phosphates that perform work for us. During very intense exercise, the energy charge of the cell goes down, i.e., the sum of ATP, ADP, and AMP goes down). This is the result of the loss of AMP via enzymatic reaction AMP>IMP+NH_3. The reader shall note this a one-way reaction, that is IMP and NH_3 cannot be used to make AMP and therefore increase the energy charge of the cell. Once AMP is lost it takes a considerable amount of time to restore the energy charge of the cell because AMP has to be synthesized De Novo (New) from Adenine (Hancock, Brault, and Terjung 2006). Additionally, acidosis as that caused by lactic acid accumulation stimulates the enzyme that breaks down AMP named AMP deaminase. This further supports a role of very intense exercise reducing the energy charge of the cell and requiring a significant amount of time for resynthesis of AMP. However, although research is scant, it would be logical that the energy charge of the cell could be enhanced and preserved through training.

KEY POINTS

1. The initiation of muscle contraction at the level of skeletal muscle occurs at activation of the sarcolemma (muscle cell membrane). Once activated the impulse travels to the T-tubule system and causes the release of Ca^{2+}.
2. The Ca^{2+} then binds to troponin and causes tropomyosin to move off of the myosin binding sites on actin so that myosin can bind.
3. The myosin head, cocked due to the breakdown of ATP, binds to the binding site on actin.
4. The myosin head contracts pulling shortening actin.
5. This process happens many times for many myosin heads and the whole muscle shortens due to the events previously listed.

4 Nervous System

Three portions of the Nervous System are extremely important for Amateur Wrestling. They are the motor system, the sympathetic Nervous System, and the parasympathetic Nervous System. The motor system sends impulses from the brain to the muscle and initiates muscle contraction. The sympathetic Nervous System allows for the activation of the body's systemic "fight or flight" reaction which prepares the body for "fight or flight" by a number of mechanisms, one of which is mobilizing energy stores and vasodilating the pre-capillary sphincters of skeletal muscle capillary beds (via epinephrine release). The parasympathetic Nervous System is called the "rest and digest" portion of the Nervous System and is important in the recovery from wrestling training and matches. The most important cell in the Nervous System is the neuron, while neuroglial cells provide a supporting role.

The Nervous System is very important when talking about athletic training and physiology. First, the Nervous System connects to the muscles and causes the muscles to contract as a result of conscious effort. Second, the sympathetic division of the autonomic Nervous System along with the hormones secreted from the adrenal medulla and adrenal cortex acts to cause a "fight or flight" reaction which prepares and engages bodies in times of stress such as training and wrestling matches. Third, the parasympathetic Nervous System is very important in recovery from training; it is called the "rest and digest" portion of the autonomic Nervous System. The overall organization of the Nervous System can be broken down into the Central Nervous System, the brain and spinal cord, and the Peripheral Nervous System which is everything else (Table 4.1). Within the Peripheral Nervous System, it can be broken down into the Somatic Nervous System which deals with the Skeletal Muscles and the Autonomic Nervous System which deals with the Cardiac Muscle, Smooth Muscle, and Glands. Additionally, further subcategories are Motor Nervous System and Sensory Nervous System. The Motor Nervous System is involved in sending

---

TABLE 4.1

Organization of the Nervous System

Central Nervous System	Peripheral Nervous System
Brain	Peripheral nerves
Spinal cord	A. Autonomic (motor and sensory)
	1. Cardiac muscle
	2. Smooth muscle
	3. Glands
	B. Somatic nervous system (motor and sensory)
	1. Skeletal muscle

conscious impulses to the muscles with voluntary effort while the Sensory Nervous System usually receives sensory input and propagates the impulse up to the Central Nervous System for evaluation.

MOTOR IMPULSES

When we are interested in contracting a muscle which is a common occurrence during amateur wrestling, we must make conscious efforts. The impulse is first initiated in the Pre-Frontal Cortex which is located in the frontal lobe of the cerebral cortex. It then goes to the Primary Motor Cortex which is just anterior or in front of the midline of the brain going front to back. Then the impulse goes down the brain stem to the spinal cord and then out the spinal cord at a level corresponding to the level of the limb, etc. that the person is trying to contract. Additionally, impulses at the same time are directed to the cerebellum, located at the posterior of the brain. These impulses are then evaluated to coordinate the muscle contraction at the level of the cerebellum. From the cerebellum, impulses leave and go down the brain stem out the spinal cord and help coordinate muscle contractions that are occurring as a direct result of the impulses originally generated in the Pre-Frontal Cortex.

THE NEURON

In addition to the physiology of an impulse involved in a voluntary contraction, it would be a good idea to know about the basic functional physiology of the Nervous System. The Neuron is the basic functional unit of the Nervous System. It is composed of Dendrites which receive impulses from other Neurons, a cell body for which the Dendrites are connected to and that house the nucleus. Further, there is a long axon which carries the impulse down the neuron to the axon terminals, and these axon terminals then connect or synapse with other neurons or connect to the muscle cell membrane. So impulses are initiated at the Dendrites, go through the cell body, are propagated down the axon, and leave the neuron through the axon terminals, usually to go to another neuron. In the case of a Motor Neuron, Neuron is connected to a muscle cell. This connection to the muscle cell is called the Motor End Plate. When the impulse reaches the end of the Motor Neuron it usually causes an action potential on the sarcolemma or muscle cell membrane. The neuron at the Neuromuscular Junction does this by taking up Ca^{2+}; when it takes up Ca^{2+} it then releases the neurotransmitter acetylcholine into the neuromuscular junction. The acetylcholine then binds to the muscle cell membrane and causes an action potential in the muscle cell which is propagated throughout the cell by the T-tubule system within the muscle cell leading to the events of muscle contraction. An interesting aside: neurons of the brain prefer to use glucose as fuel; however, they can run on ketones in the case of starvation. What is uncertain is how long it takes to be able to run on ketones as efficiently as glucose. Thus, there is likely a time lag between optimal cognitive efficiency on glucose and optimal cognitive efficiency while utilizing ketones; if in fact your brain can use ketones as effectively as glucose.

NEUROGLIAL CELLS

There are four types of neuroglial cells. Astrocytes which form metabolic and structural support cells and are often connected to capillaries and form the blood–brain barrier, Microglial cells which remove debris and can attack microbes, Ependymal cells which cover surfaces and line cavities as epithelial cells, and Oligodendrocytes which form the myelin within the central Nervous System and help to hold nerve fibers together (Colbert, Anckney, and Lee 2020).

KEY POINTS

Initiation of muscle contraction:

1. Nervous impulses are initiated in the pre-frontal cortex.
2. The impulses then travel to the primary motor cortex near the middle of the cerebrum on both sides of the corpus callosum.
3. The impulse then goes down through the thalamus and some of it branches off to the cerebellum for fine motor tuning.
4. Once through the thalamus, the impulse travels far away down the motor neuron to the level of the muscle to contract.
5. Once to the axon terminal that connects nerve to muscle, Ca^{2+} is taken up by the axon terminal and there is the release of the neurotransmitter acetylcholine.
6. Once acetylcholine binds to the muscle cell membrane, an action potential in the muscle cell membrane occurs. This triggers the events in skeletal muscle leading to muscle contraction.
7. The neuron is the primary cell of the Nervous System and consists of dendrites, a cell body, an axon, and axon terminals.
8. The neuroglial cells are support cells of the Nervous System and support the function of the neurons.

5 The Cardiovascular System

The heart, blood vessels, and lymphatic vessels form the cardiovascular system. Cardiac Output (the amount of blood the heart pumps per minute) is an important concept for Amateur Wrestling. It is made up of the Stroke Volume, the amount of blood the heart pumps per beat, and the Heart Rate which is the number of beats per minute. Cardiac Output is a major determinant of VO_2peak/max, or the amount of oxygen that can be delivered by the heart and lungs and taken up by the cells and utilized during exercise. The Arteriovenous Oxygen Difference (A-VO_2 diff) is the other major determinant of VO_2peak/max and is dependent on extraction of oxygen out of the blood at the tissue level. Factors which influence A-VO_2 difference are capillarity, and mitochondrial size, and number.

The heart and all the blood vessels of the body make up the cardiovascular system. The heart is a four-chambered organ with right and left atria and right and left ventricles. The atria are involved in delivering the blood to the ventricles and the ventricles are involved in the delivery of the blood to the lungs and to the systemic circulation. The circulatory system starts at the largest artery in the body of the aorta. The oxygenated blood is pumped from the left ventricle through the aorta to the systemic circulation. From the aorta the oxygenated blood goes to the arteries, the arterioles which have a muscular precapillary sphincter, and to the capillaries where oxygen/nutrient and CO_2/waste exchange occur. After this exchange at the capillary level, deoxygenated blood is returned to the heart by way of the venules, veins, and then great veins. Once the blood reaches the great veins (Superior and Inferior Vena Cava) the blood is then dumped into the right atrium. After the blood is dumped into the right atrium, the blood goes into the right ventricle, and the right ventricle then pumps the blood through the pulmonary artery to the lungs. After the blood goes to the lungs, it comes back to the left atrium and then left ventricle and is then pumped to the systemic circulation as discussed above.

The formed elements are the red blood cells, white blood cells, and platelets/thrombocytes as well as the plasma. In a normal individual, the formed elements make up about 45% of the blood while plasma makes up the other 55% of the blood. Leukocytes and platelets make up less than 1% of the formed elements (Figure 5.1).

Plasma contains the proteins albumin, fibrinogen, and globulins. Plasma is primarily water in addition to these proteins. Red blood cells contain the protein hemoglobin which has binding sites for oxygen. The major function of the red blood cells is to transport oxygen. The red blood cells pick up oxygen at the lungs as they go through and dump the oxygen off at the level of the tissue capillaries where the oxygen can go into the cells and be used for cellular metabolism and the production of large quantities of the energy substance called ATP in the mitochondria. Additionally, the white blood cells are cells of the immune system, and they are

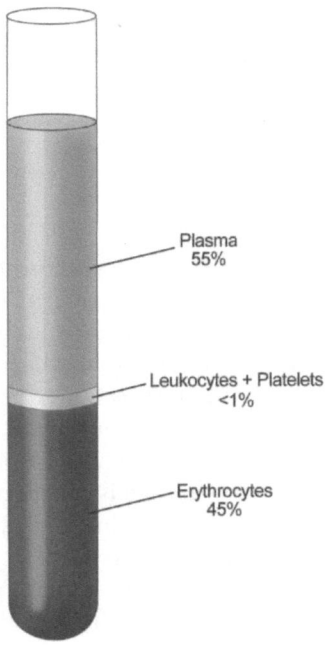

Plasma
55%

Leukocytes + Platelets
<1%

Erythrocytes
45%

FIGURE 5.1 Formed elements.

the defense system of the body against foreign invaders. The platelets are involved in blood clotting and quantitatively a very small portion of the formed elements. Together the white blood cells are also called leukocytes, and platelets make up less than 1% of the formed elements.

One of the major functions of the cardiovascular system is to pump blood to the tissues. This is called Cardiac Output (Q) and is expressed in L/min. Cardiac output is equal to stroke volume × heart rate ($Q = SV \times HR$). Stroke volume is the amount of blood pumped per beat, and heart rate is the number of beats per minute. Cardiac output is about 5 L/min in most individuals and can increase to 25 L/min during extreme exercise. Another important measure for exercise is the maximal oxygen consumption (VO_2max). VO_2max is calculated by cardiac output × A-VO_2diff. VO_2max is the maximal amount of oxygen one can use at the cellular level and that these can be delivered to the tissue by cardiovascular system. A-VO_2diff is difference in the oxygen content on the arterial side of the capillary bed relative to the venous side of the capillary bed and is a measure of tissue extraction of oxygen. Much of A-VO_2 diff is dependent on the number of capillaries, the number and function of the mitochondria at the subcellular level and the demand of the cell for oxygen, i.e., relative and absolute intensity of exercise. Interestingly one factor that will influence VO_2max is plasma volume. Relatively speaking, the greater the plasma volume, the greater the delivery of oxygen to the tissues. This is due to the Frank-Starling Mechanism of the Heart, which states the heart will pump the blood that is returned to it. The greater the plasma volume, the greater the blood returned to the heart and therefore the greater the stroke volume, cardiac output, and likely VO_2. This is exactly the reason that dehydration results in impaired exercise performance. Much of the fluid that is lost due to dehydration comes from the plasma space. When the plasma is lost, this decreases the fluid that is returned to the heart and stroke volume, and the cardiac output goes down. Likewise, one of the important adaptations to exercise is the gain in plasma volume that occurs as a result of exercise training (Wilmore and Costill 1994). Albumin concentrations in blood are a measure of protein nutrition. Low albumin concentrations are indicative of poor protein nutrition. Since plasma volume depends on albumin concentrations and plasma volume is a major determinant of VO_2peak, the loss of plasma albumin due to protein malnutrition could be a factor in a decline in VO_2 peak in malnutrition due to too severe protein energy restriction.

KEY POINTS

1. The heart, all of the blood vessels, and the lymphatic system make up the cardiovascular system.
2. The heart pumps oxygenated blood systemically and deoxygenated blood to the lungs for oxygenation.
3. Oxygen/Nutrient exchange and CO_2/Waste exchange happen at the level of the capillaries the blood flow into which is regulated by precapillary sphincters.
4. Fifty-five percent (approximately) of the blood is made up of plasma, 45% is made up of red blood cells, and less than 1% is made up of platelets and leukocytes.
5. The pumping capacity of the heart to the tissues is Cardiac Output. Cardiac Output is equal to the amount of blood pumped per beat, and the heart rate is the number of beats per minute (CO = SV × HR).
6. The ability to inspire oxygen, deliver it to the tissues, and the uptake and use of oxygen by the tissues are termed VO_2peak. VO_2peak = Cardiac Output × A-VO_2diff. Cardiac Output is the heart's pumping ability, and A-VO_2diff is also termed extraction and use at the cellular level.

6 Gastrointestinal Tract

The gastrointestinal tract is the path from mouth to anus also called the alimentary canal. It is important for the wrestler from the standpoint of digestion and absorption of food and water. Protein digestion begins in the stomach, and absorption of amino acids occurs in the small intestine. Carbohydrate digestion begins in the mouth with salivary amylase but bypasses digestion in the stomach and gets further digested and absorbed in the small intestine. Lipid digestion occurs primarily in the small intestine and the majority (about 2/3rdtwo-thirds) of the lipid is absorbed by the lymphatic system. Water and electrolyte absorption occur primarily in the small intestine, while the large intestine is a storage depot for waste but can absorb and secrete water out of and into the waste. Water and electrolyte losses from single athletic practice and two a days can be substantial and may not be able to replace in the hours prior to the next practice. Additionally, at higher exercise intensities there are proportionally greater electrolyte losses than at lower intensities, suggesting that high-intensity exercise promotes greater electrolyte losses than low low-intensity exercise.

DIGESTION

Clearly, a book on Nutrition for Wrestling should have a chapter on how to digest the constituents of foods and fluids. After ingestion at the level of the mouth, food and fluid that are composed of long chain carbohydrate (polysaccharide) undergo the digestion by salivary amylase which partially breaks down these carbohydrates. The food and fluid then travel down the esophagus to the stomach. The stomach is a place for initial protein digestion and some fluid absorption but not much. Hydrochloric acid which is highly acidic is secreted in the stomach. This hydrochloric acid provides an environment for the gastric (stomach) enzyme pepsin to be active, and this enzyme starts the breakdown of proteins. Not much digestion of lipids (fats) or carbohydrates occurs in the stomach, and this will occur in the small intestine. The partially digested proteins as well as carbohydrates and lipids then pass through the pyloric sphincter to the small intestine. The rate of passage of these nutrients to the small intestine is dictated by the energy (caloric) density of the stomach's contents. That is, the more energy dense the food, the slower the rate of gastric emptying into the small intestine and vice versa. The stomach contents that pass into the duodenum of the small intestine then begin the process of further digestion and then absorption from the small intestine primarily into the circulation (or blood stream). The digestion of proteins further occurs in the small intestine, and the protein is acted on by pancreatic secretion of proteolytic enzymes. The pancreas is a vital organ (we can't live without) which produces key hormones in glucose metabolism and also secretes key enzymes in protein, carbohydrate, and lipid breakdown. The proteins and smaller members of the protein family are then broken down into amino acids, the building blocks of protein. Additionally, the brush border of the epithelial cells of the small intestine contain enzymes that break down dipeptides (two amino acids) into the constituent amino acids. With regard to carbohydrate breakdown, pancreatic amylase breaks down maltose and other small polymers of glucose down to glucose. Then the intestinal brush border has enzymes to convert disaccharides to monosaccharides which prior to getting beyond the second portion of the small intestine called the jejunum (duodenum, jejunum, and ileum comprise the small intestine). The breakdown of lipids primarily occurs in the small intestine by the secretion of pancreatic lipase which breaks down triglycerides (three fatty acids and a glycerol) to three fatty acids and a glycerol molecule. Typically, this is with the help of bile which is secreted from the gall bladder and bile helps to emulsify or make the lipid easier to break down.

ABSORPTION OF PROTEINS, CARBOHYDRATES, AND LIPIDS

The duodenum and jejunum of the small intestine have folds which increase the surface area of these portions of the small intestine by about 20 times or 20-fold. This greatly increases the surface area. These folds are called Villi. The Villi come complete with blood vessels and a central lymph vessel called the central lacteal. The amino acids from protein, the monosaccharides from carbohydrate, and the fatty acids and glycerol are taken up by the Villi. The amino acids and monosaccharides go into the capillaries of the Villi, while most of the fat goes into the Central Lacteal of the Villi (Guyton and Hall 2006; Table 6.1).

FACTORS REGULATING GASTRIC EMPTYING AND INTESTINAL ABSORPTION OF INGESTED FLUIDS

Both gastric emptying and intestinal absorption must occur prior to a fluid being absorbed into the blood stream. The composition of the ingested fluid will affect the gastric emptying and intestinal absorption as well as the retention of the absorbed fluid within the body. Major factors regulating the gastric emptying rate from stomach to small intestine are the energy density of the ingested fluid and

TABLE 6.1
Regions and Functions of the Gastrointestinal Tract

Region of the Gastrointestinal Tract	Generalized Function
Stomach	Digestion of proteins
Small intestine	Digestion and absorption of carbohydrates and lipids and absorption of proteins and water
Large intestine	Absorption of and secretion of water into the feces, synthesis of vitamin K

the osmolality of the ingested fluid. The more energy (kcal or kJ/ml) dense the solution the slower the gastric emptying rate, and the higher the osmotic pressure of the ingested fluid the slower the gastric emptying rate. Thus, for maximal rates of gastric emptying the carbohydrate content must be low or moderately low for maximal gastric emptying (0%–6% carbohydrate concentration). Factors that add to increase the osmolality and slow the rate of gastric emptying are things such as a high electrolyte concentration. For example, chicken noodle soup which would be excellent in the long run (many hours to days) for rehydration because of the high sodium concentration likely leads to a very slow gastric emptying rate in the short term. Because of the high Na^+ concentration (i.e., particle number per mL or kg of fluid). Also, the carbohydrate concentration needs to be adequate to maximize carbohydrate oxidation during exercise. So, there are four variables the athlete/coach must consider when selecting a rehydration solution. Will it rehydrate the athlete quickly, will it maximize carbohydrate storage, will it maximize carbohydrate oxidation during exercise, and will it lead to long-term rehydration. As discussed in subsequent sections one rehydration solution may be good for one situation but not so good for another situation. Another variable which regulates the rate of gastric emptying is the volume of ingested fluid. Generally speaking, the greater the volume up to 800 mL (Costill and Saltin 1974), the greater the rate of gastric emptying. An additional factor that dictates whether a solution empties and is absorbed into the circulation is the temperature of the fluid. Costill and Saltin (1974) showed that cool solutions result in faster gastric emptying than warmer solutions. In contrast, when both gastric emptying and intestinal absorption are taken into account with the use of the deuterium oxide tracer methodology, hot solutions get into the circulation at a similar rate as cold solutions (Lambert and Maughan 1992), suggesting greater intestinal absorption of warm solutions. One potentially important factor that has not been examined is the ability of the ingested fluid to cool the body during exercise. It is likely that the ingestion of cool fluids will have some effect on keeping the body temperature down during exercise. Due to the effect on body temperature it would behoove the athlete to take in cold fluids during exercise. The optimal temperature fluid to be ingested at rest (when body temperature is a minor factor) would appear not to matter (Lambert and Maughan 1992). With regard to fluid delivery to the circulation (Evans, Shirreffs, and Maughan 2011) and fluid retention (Evans, Shirreffs, and Maughan 2009), solutions which contain 52–100 mmol/L sodium and about 2%–10% glucose have shown to be optimal. The high sodium concentration and adequate glucose concentration optimize sodium/glucose cotransport across the intestinal epithelial cell wall and absorption of water by osmosis into the circulatory system. The key game you are playing with your oral rehydration solution is how much muscle glycogen are you going to synthesize relative to your ability to rapidly rehydrate. A 0%–2% glucose solution will allow rapid rehydration but the trade-off is that muscle glycogen resynthesis rate will be much slower than if a 6% or 10% carbohydrate solution is ingested. Additionally, a high sodium concentration (52–100 mmol/L) and high volume of ingestion 150% of what was lost is necessary for optimal rehydration in the days after high sweat losses.

ABSORPTION OF WATER AND ELECTROLYTES

Water and electrolytes pretty much pass through the stomach to the small intestine without being absorbed, and once in the small intestine, the absorption of these vital nutrients begins in the duodenum and the jejunum. Interestingly, Jeukendrup et al. (2009) found that the addition of glucose to water at a concentration of 3% was more effective than water alone with regard to the appearance of the solution in the circulation after ingestion. This was the case as the appearance of deuterium oxide added to a solution after ingestion is indicative of both gastric emptying and intestinal absorption. The addition of glucose at a concentration of 6% and 9% resulted in slower appearance in the circulation than that of the 3% concentration of glucose. The authors eluded to data which suggest that the glucose is essential for glucose and sodium cotransport and the osmosis of water after the cotransport of glucose and sodium. Thus, the addition to of glucose to plain water at a low concentration is an important consideration for maximizing fluid delivery to the circulation.

EFFECTS OF EXERCISE ON FLUID AND ELECTROLYTE LOSSES

Professional basketball players have been found to lose considerable amounts of fluid during a game: from 1 to 4.6 L and do not completely rehydrate before subsequent games (Ostenberg et al.). This is indicated by the fact that 52% of the players had a urine-specific gravity (USG) above 1.020 μg/L, indicating hypohydration prior to the game. This problem of preexercise hypohydration does not only seem to be a problem in professional athletes but also a problem in high-school athletes as Cleary et al. (2012) reported that 25% of high-school female volleyball players in their study came to practice in the hypohydrated state with a USG greater or equal to 1.020 μgs/L. In this study, an educational intervention was not sufficient to increase prepractice hydration levels nor was a prescribed hydration intervention.

Godek et al. (2008) studied the Philadelphia Eagles football team over the course of a week during two a day practices during team camp. Interestingly when players practiced for 4.5 hours/day, sweat sodium losses were 2 g up to a maximum of 30 g/day (one player). The authors concluded that it would take close to 65 L of a carbohydrate electrolyte beverage to replace sodium lost in sweat for the player that lost 30 g. Also, for backs and receivers, linebackers and quarterbacks and linemen weight loss replaced with fluid was 66% of the total volume lost. This means there was a 34% deficit in with regard to fluid replacement, and clearly the athlete would be in the hypohydrated state.

Baker et al. (2019) reported that when exercise intensity was taken from 45% to 65% of VO_2 max for 90 minutes, sweat Na^+ losses increased 150%, and sweat Cl^- losses increased even more. Sweat Na^+ losses were about 1.5 g and sweat Cl^- losses were 2.4 g, while K^+ losses were about 1.9 g. These subjects were not heat acclimatized. The sweat Na^+ losses would require the consumption of about 3.25 L of the sports drink while the potassium losses would require the consumption of 4.5 bananas in addition to the fluid that was lost. Little data are available for the sweat Na^+, sweat K^+, and sweat Cl^- losses during high-intensity exercise of an intermittent nature such as wrestling. Thus, the greater the intensity of the exercise the greater the electrolyte losses. It could be hypothesized that the sweat electrolyte losses would be very high because of the high-intensity nature of wrestling interspersed with rest periods, i.e., like a wrestling practice.

O'Neal et al. (2014) reported that a one hour run in ~20.0°C temperature resulted in the loss of 1.353 L of sweat as a result of the run. Most runners were euhydrated (USG below 1.020 µgs/L at 12 or 24 hours post run when both genders were included. At 12 hours USG was 1.025 µgs/L in men who consumed 171% of what they lost and 1.014 in women who consumed 268% of sweat losses. These investigators suggested that USG measurements are inexpensive to detect athletes who have problems with hydration strategies as a result of a poor perception of fluid losses during exercise.

KEY POINTS

1. Proteins are primarily broken down in the stomach and the amino acids absorbed in the small intestine.
2. Carbohydrate breakdown begins in the mouth and continues in the small intestine, while absorption of the monosaccharides happens in the small intestine.
3. Fat breakdown is primarily in the small intestine, while fatty acids and glycerol are primarily absorbed by the central lacteal of the lymphatic system.
4. Absorption of water and electrolytes primarily occurs in the duodenum and jejunum of the small intestine.
5. The athlete/coach needs to determine the priorities for fluid/carbohydrate/ electrolyte replacement with post-weigh in food and fluid consumption; i.e., rapid fluid replacement and/or rapid muscle glycogen resynthesis and/ or long-term rehydration.
6. Fluid and electrolyte losses are substantial in athletes, and many times fluid consumption cannot keep up with water and electrolyte losses.
7. Increasing exercise intensity, recently, has been shown to cause a greater than expected increase in electrolyte losses. This should be taken into consideration in intense intermittent sports such as amateur wrestling.

7 Endocrine System

The endocrine system deals with all of the glands that produce hormones and the hormones themselves. The hypothalamus is considered the "Commander and Chief" while the pituitary is considered the "master gland" and is usually under the control of the hypothalamus. Hormones are classified by their mechanism of action: ; generally there are two distinct mechanisms of action, one is to bind to cell surface and cause the release of a second messenger within the cell, and then cause a cascade of reactions leading to a change in metabolism. The other mechanism of action is that the hormones pass through the cell membrane and bind to a binding protein and then interact with the DNA to alter gene expression and then they alter metabolism. The posterior pituitary releases oxytocin and antidiuretic hormone (ADH) directly into the circulation. The anterior pituitary releases stimulating hormones that go to a gland and cause release of the hormone of interest from the gland of interest, and the hormone then circulates in blood, binds to the target tissue, and causes changes in metabolism. The adrenal medulla releases epinephrine and norepinephrine which have strong effects on cardiovascular function and the "fight or flight" response, while the adrenal cortex releases cortisol which is also active in the "fight or flight" response and stimulates muscle protein breakdown and gluconeogenesis (the making of new glucose from a non-glucose source). It is also important in the release of aldosterone which primarily leads to Na^+ and reabsorption in the kidney. The pancreatic hormones are insulin and glucagon. Insulin results in a lowering of blood glucose as a result of glucose uptake by cells while glucagon acts to breakdown liver glycogen to glucose thus raising blood glucose concentrations. The major sex hormones are testosterone which increases muscle mass, estrogen, and progesterone, both of which the latter two stimulate the development of secondary female sex characteristics. The thyroid secretes T3 and T4, the hormones that stimulate thermogenic metabolism in addition to calcitonin which lowers blood calcium. The parathyroid gland acts to secrete hormones that raise blood calcium.

Hormones are blood-borne substances released from one organ that circulate and stimulate biochemical reactions in another organ or organs (Guyton and Hall 2006). The hypothalamus is said to be the "commander in chief" of the endocrine system is the hormones and all of the organs and tissues involved in their release and uptake. The pituitary is said to be "the master gland" since it releases all of the stimulating hormones which stimulate the effector organs, and under most conditions, the pituitary is under the control of the hypothalamus. The hypothalamus receives input by the circulating levels of end hormones and under negative feedback homeostatic control mechanisms regulates the secretion of releasing hormones that go down to the pituitary. The pituitary will then put out stimulating hormones that are directed by the hypothalamus, which go to the effector organs and cause the release of the primary circulating hormone that goes to the blood and binds to target organs and DNA and effects metabolism or the biochemistry of the body. Two hormones are secreted directly by the posterior pituitary (Neurohypophysis) into the circulation, namely Oxytocin and ADH. All other hormones have a Releasing Hormone released by the hypothalamus that goes to the pituitary and cause the release of a Stimulating Hormone which acts at the effector organ to cause Primary Hormone release.

HORMONE ACTION

Generally speaking, there are two ways in which hormone action takes place. The first (made of amino acids, peptides, or proteins) is binding to the cell membrane receptor, causing a conformational change in that receptor and causing the liberation of a Second Messenger within the cytosol of the cell. Quite often this second messenger is Cyclic Adenosine Monophoshate (AMP) which is made from Adenosine Triphosphate (ATP) utilizing the enzyme Adenylate Cyclase. Once liberated inside the cell, the Cyclic AMP causes a cascade of events that lead to things like the breakdown of liver glycogen to blood glucose and the liberation of fatty acids and glycerol from triglycerides in a fat cell.

The other way in which hormones, especially those comprised of steroids (testosterone, estrogen, and progesterone in addition to T3 and T4) act, because they are lipid soluble, is by diffusing through the cell membrane and binding to DNA. After they bind to DNA, they cause gene expression (transcription) and ultimately protein synthesis (translation).

THE HORMONES OF THE ADRENAL GLAND

The adrenal gland has two important areas from which it secretes hormones. One is the adrenal medulla and the other is the adrenal cortex. Both the adrenal medulla and the adrenal cortex are involved in the "fight or flight" response. The adrenal medulla secretes epinephrine (adrenaline) and norepinephrine (noradrenaline) while the adrenal cortex secretes the glucocorticoid cortisol and the mineralocorticoids, primarily aldosterone. Epinephrine has a myriad of effects, like stimulating the breakdown of glycogen in muscle and liver cells, increasing the strength of contraction of the heart, and liberating fatty acids and glycerol from triglycerides at the adipocyte. Also, epinephrine acts to cause dilation of the precapillary sphincters of the arterioles in skeletal muscle capillary beds allowing for increased perfusion, i.e., blood flow to skeletal muscle during exercise. Norepinephrine generally increases heart rate and causes vasoconstriction all over the body. As opposed to the hormonal control of the release of epinephrine and norepinephrine from the adrenal medulla it is under direct sympathetic nervous system control. That is, when "fight or flight" situation arises, the nervous system stimulates the release of epinephrine and norepinephrine from the adrenal medulla.

Cortisol is released from the adrenal cortex. Being a glucocorticoid, it acts to stimulate gluconeogenesis in the liver (the formation of new glucose form noncarbohydrate sources). High cortisol levels will degrade muscle protein to amino acids for gluconeogenic precursors (subunits that can be used to make new glucose). There are no known effects of cortisol on the fat cell or on the degradation of liver glycogen. Cortisol secretion by the adrenal cortex is under the control of adrenocorticotrophic hormone (ACTH) which is secreted by the pituitary in response to corticotropin releasing hormone (CRH) release from the hypothalamus. Aldosterone (a mineralo-corticoid) acts to cause reabsorption of Na^+ in the kidney and secretion of K^+ into the kidney tubules for release into the urine. Quantitatively, the reabsorption of Na^+ is extremely important as water follows Na^+ by osmosis. Therefore, we retain water when aldosterone levels rise. Aldosterone concentrations in plasma are under the complex control of the Renin–Angiotensin system. Briefly, renin is released by the kidney in response to low blood pressure (which is caused by decreased blood vol-ume). Renin goes to the liver and renin substrate is converted to angiotensin I. The angiotensin I then goes to the lungs and is converted to angiotensin II by Angiotensin Converting Enzyme (ACE). Angiotensin II has potent vasoconstrictor properties and as well goes to the liver to stimulate aldosterone secretion by the adrenal cortex. In dehydration both the vasoconstriction and the secretion of aldosterone are important for an increase in effective plasma volume and blood pressure which decreased as a result of dehydration.

THE PRIMARY HORMONES OF THE PANCREAS

Insulin, glucagon, and somatostatin are the primary hormones of the pan-creas. Insulin's primary role is to allow for the uptake of glucose from the blood into the cells. Most of the insulin stimulated glucose uptake is in skeletal muscle (85%; Defronzo et al. 1981). In other instances, insulin stimulated glucose uptake is in liver and adipose or fat cells. Insulin is also involved in amino acid uptake into muscle cells. Insulin is often perceived as a bad hormone due to its high lev-els of insulin resistance. However, the high level of insulin *is in response* to the insulin resistance, not the cause of the insulin resistance. Insulin resistance is the inability of normal amounts of insulin to allow glucose primarily into the muscle cells resulting in the rise of blood glucose, i.e., hyperglycemia occurs as a result of this. Hyperglycemia has a number of chronic problems associated with it; Type II Diabetes being one of these problems. Let it be said that insulin is not in and of itself a bad hormone and clearly does not "make you fat". It has little negative effect on metabolic rate and may stimulate metabolic rate by stimulating glucose uptake and glycolysis. It does have an effect of reducing fat liberation, but without an effect on metabolic rate, this in and of itself will not "make you fat". Additionally, carbohy-drate gets a bad reputation because it raises the insulin levels. Clearly, carbohydrate balance (carbohydrate intake vs. carbohydrate use) in the muscle and fat balance (fat intake vs. fat use) in the muscle are important considerations when determining whether insulin resistance will occur.

Glucagon is an important hormone that counteracts the effects of insulin. That is glucagon causes the breakdown of liver glycogen to blood glucose. In contrast to insu-lin, however, there are no receptors for glucagon in the skeletal muscle. Glucagon has no known effect on the fat cell. Glucagon also increases the rate of gluconeogenesis in the liver. Insulin and Glucagon are under control by blood glucose concentrations. When blood glucose concentrations go up, insulin is secreted in negative feedback fashion to reduce blood glucose concentrations. When blood glucose concentrations are low, on the other hand, glucagon is increased and the blood glucose concentration is increased in negative feedback fashion to maintain blood glucose. Clearly, the ratio of insulin to glucagon is an important factor in the level of blood glucose at any one time.

TESTOSTERONE

The male sex hormone testosterone is secreted minimally in childhood, increased secretion in adolescent boys and the early 20s, and a there is a steady decline in testosterone from about the age of 40 until death. A major effect of testosterone is to increase muscle mass, and this is the reason for the large increase in muscle mass seen in adolescents and the early 20s. Interestingly, testosterone concentrations go down in plasma with overtraining (Flynn, Pizza, and Brolinson 1997; Kageta et al. 2016). This clearly is not a good adaptation for athletes wanting to build and repair muscle on a daily basis. Therefore, for this and other reasons, the monitoring of overtraining and the implementation of drug testing would seem to be of paramount importance.

ESTROGEN AND PROGESTERONE

The female sex hormones estrogen and progesterone are secreted at relatively low concentrations in the female until menses or the first menstruation around the time of puberty at which time these hormones increase greatly and help in the development of female sex characteristics and prepare the woman for child birth. These hormones remain relatively stable until the time of menopause at about age 50 when both of these hormones drop drastically.

THE THYROID HORMONES

The thyroid hormones T3 and T4 are very important for energy metabolism. Most of the T4 gets converted into T3 in the tissues, and therefore, T3 is considered the most important of these two with regard to energy metabolism. Along with stimulating energy metabolism these two hormones act to increase thermogenesis or heat production. Thyroid hormones stimulate protein synthesis, increase the amount and activity of enzymes involved in cellular metabolism, and increase the size and number of mitochondria in almost all cells (Guyton and Hall 2006). It seems apparent; therefore, that having normal thyroid function would appear important to staving off obesity. Thyroid hormone release from the thyroid is under the control of thyroid stimulating hormone release from the pituitary and under the control and the pituitary release of TSH is under the control of TRH release from the hypothalamus. Like most hormones this is under negative feedback control.

CALCITONIN

The third hormone released from the Thyroid is Calcitonin. This hormone is released in response to high blood Ca^{2+} levels. The action of Calcitonin is to reduce blood Ca^{2+} levels by a number of means.

THE PARATHYROID GLAND

The parathyroid gland acts to secrete parathyroid hormone which acts to increase blood Ca^{2+} concentrations by causing the degradation of bones and to raise blood Ca^{2+} concentrations in a time when blood Ca^{2+} may be low.

ACUTE EXERCISE RESPONSES TO SELECTED HORMONES

As a result of exercise, norepinephrine and epinephrine increase. Norepinephrine increases at about 50% of VO_2max while Epinephrine increases at about 60%–70% of VO_2max (Wilmore and Costill 1994). Clearly these are involved in the "fight or flight" response. A major effect of epinephrine is that it causes lipolysis at the fat cell lysing triglyceride into free fatty acids and glycerol. The free fatty acids can be oxidized in muscle for fuel. During prolonged exercise of moderate intensity (60% of VO_2peak), both epinephrine and norepinephrine gradually creep up and during 3 hours of exercise will peak at 3 hours of exercise. Cortisol increases at 60% of VO_2max (Jacks et al. 2002) and is also involved in the "fight or flight" response. During prolonged exercise cortisol increases until about the first 30 minutes of exercise and then drops dramatically after that.

The primary regulators of the blood glucose concentration glucagon and insulin also undergo changes with the exercise. In untrained subjects' glucagon goes up dramatically at the onset of exercise, while in trained individuals this increase is gradual and less than half the increase as in the untrained individual. Insulin declines dramatically at about 30 minutes of exercise in the untrained individual, while the decrease in the trained individual happens at about the same time but is about half of that as the trained individual (Wilmore and Costill 1994). The rise of glucagon and the lowering of insulin allow for the mobilization of glucose from the liver, and the reduction in insulin also allows for the mobilization of free fatty acids from the fat cell. Little increase in growth hormone is seen until 60 minutes of exercise where it goes up to a great extent.

As plasma volume goes down, aldosterone concentrations gradually rise, and this leads to the retention of sodium and water.

Chronic changes in resting testosterone and cortisol concentrations can be considered an indicator of overtraining syndrome with testosterone declining dramatically and cortisol increasing, thus altering the anabolic to catabolic hormone ratio.

In summary, the hormonal changes that occur during exercise result in the mobilization of fuel stores and the protection of blood glucose concentrations so that they stay near normal until the body runs out of liver glycogen. Additionally, the reduction in plasma volume triggers aldosterone secretion for improved retention of sodium and water. Overtraining leads to a decline in the testosterone concentration and an increase in the cortisol concentration.

KEY POINTS

1. The hypothalamus is considered the "Commander-in-Chief" gland while the pituitary is considered the "Master Gland".

2. Hormones work basically in two ways: (1) Bind to a cell surface receptor and cause a cascade of events, (2) Diffuse through the cell membrane and bind to the DNA and cause changes in gene expression.

3. The adrenal gland is broken down into the Medulla and the Cortex. The adrenal medulla secretes epinephrine and norepinephrine while the adrenal cortex secretes cortisol and mineralocorticoids.

4. The primary hormones of the pancreas are insulin and glucagon. Insulin lowers blood glucose by causing primarily skeletal muscle to take up blood glucose. Glucagon increases blood glucose by causing the liver to degrade liver glycogen into blood glucose.

5. The primary sex hormone in men is Testosterone, while in women Estrogen and Progesterone are the primary sex hormones. These hormones cause secondary sex characteristics in men such as deepened voice and an increase in muscle mass, and in women Estrogen and Progesterone cause the development of breast tissue and regulation of the menstrual cycle.

6. The thyroid gland secretes three hormones: T3 and T4 which act to speed up the metabolic rate. A third hormone secreted by the thyroid is Calcitonin which causes a reduction in blood calcium levels.

7. The parathyroid gland secretes Parathyroid hormone which raises blood calcium levels by causing the bones to give up some of their calcium.

8. Hormonal changes that occur during exercise are meant to maintain blood glucose concentrations and mobilize fuel for exercise as well as maintain plasma volume.

9. A reduction in resting testosterone and an increase in resting cortisol concentrations accompany chronic, high-volume, high-intensity training.

8 Muscle Fiber Types

There are three major fiber types: Slow Twitch (Type I), Fast Twitch Oxidative Glycolytic (FOG) (Type IIa), and Fast Twitch Glycolytic (Type IIb) fibers. This is via staining by way of the Myosin ATPase assay (Padykula and Herman 1955; Dubowitz and Neville 1973). The myosin corresponding to these fiber types is actually on a continuum meaning that the Myosin ATPase assay is a way to force them into categories. More recent analyses include gel electrophoresis, and clearly there is a continuum from slow to fast rather than distinct delineations. Nonetheless, the Myosin ATPase method of classification has stood the test time. Slow twitch fibers have low contraction velocity, low force, and generally not very fatigable. FOG fibers have high contraction velocity, high force, and low to moderate fatigability. Fast twitch glycolytic fibers have a high contraction velocity, high force, and high fatigability. Typically, during exercise of increasing intensity, slow twitch fibers are recruited first, followed by FOG, and by fast twitch glycolytic fibers. Training can result in a fast twitch glycolytic fiber becoming a FOG fiber. Under situations of extreme endurance training a FOG fiber can become a slow twitch fiber. Based on the sum toto of all the data it does not appear that a slow twitch fiber can become a FOG fiber or a fast twitch glycolytic fiber although there have been scant reports of this occurrence (Jansson et al. 1990). Generally speaking, endurance training will increase the number of capillaries in skeletal muscle capillary beds that are used, increase the number and function of mitochondria, and increase the amount of oxidative enzymes in the skeletal muscle. These adaptations will improve arteriovenous oxygen difference one of the components of VO_2max/peak (Wilmore and Costill 1994) (Table 8.1).

PHYSIOLOGICAL AND BIOCHEMICAL BACKGROUND: MUSCLE FIBER TYPES

Clearly, if you want to train a muscle for any reason it would help to know the makeup of the muscle as well as how the muscle adapts to training. Here I will discuss the various muscle fiber types and then I will discuss their response to training. Traditionally, muscle fiber types have been broken down into three types:

TABLE 8.1
Classifications Based on Myosin ATPase Staining

	Slow Twitch (Type I)	FOG (Type IIA)	Fast Twitch (Type IIB)
Contraction velocity	Low	High	High
Force	Low	High	High
Fatigability	Low	Low–moderate	High

Slow Twitch oxidative, FOG, and Fast Twitch Glycolytic fibers (Wilmore and Costill 1994). Slow Twitch are Type I, FOG (FOGs as they are called) are Type IIa, and Fast Twitch Glycolytic are Type IIb. This is a dichotomous classification and simplistic as the myosin heavy chain amount is actually on a continuum (Trappe et al. 2015). However, for our purposes the excellent, time held, traditional, classification system will work. Slow Twitch fibers have a slow contraction speed and are not very fatigable due to their oxidative nature. FOG fibers are fast contracting but are also not fatigable. They are also red in color just like slow twitch oxidative. Fast Twitch Glycolytic are fast contracting but are very fatigable. They are white in color. The color of the fibers is reflective of the muscle oxygen carrying protein myoglobin. Fast Twitch Glycolytic and Slow Twitch Oxidative Fibers are good for endurance activities while Fast Twitch Glycolytic Fibers are good for strength and power-type activities like sprinting. The FOG fibers, however, can produce considerable strength (force) and power (force×distance/time).

MOTOR UNIT RECRUITMENT

A motor nerve, and the muscle fibers it connects to (innervates), is called a motor unit. The motor nerves vary in size from the smallest that are slow twitch oxidative, medium are FOG fibers, and fast twitch glycolytic fibers are the largest. Motor unit recruitment or engaging the different muscle fibers follows the size principle (McComas 1996). With increasing force of contraction the larger motor neurons are recruited. During low force contractions the slow twitch oxidative fibers are recruited, during higher force contractions the FOG fibers in addition to the slow twitch oxidative fibers are recruited, and during the highest force contractions the fast twitch glycolytic fibers are also recruited. So force dictates the degree of motor unit recruitment. The higher the force, the greater the number of motor units and the number of fast twitch fibers recruited. Speed of contraction has little to do with motor unit recruitment. That is, at fast contraction velocities (speeds) with little force, only slow twitch fibers are recruited (McComas 1996). Once force is increased, more motor units and the fast twitch fibers starting with the fast twitch oxidative glycolytic get recruited. Last, at maximal forces all motor units are recruited including the fast twitch glycolytic, FOG, and slow twitch oxidative fibers (Henneman 1979).

EFFECTS OF TRAINING ON MUSCLE FIBER TYPE

Endurance training can convert an FG fiber to an FOG fiber. Therefore, it makes a fatigable fiber considerably less fatigable. Long-term electrical stimulation of rat muscles has shown that an FG fiber can be converted all the way to an SO fiber (Pette et al. 1975). This may also occur with extensive long-term endurance training (McComas 1996). On the other hand there is little evidence to suggest that strength or power training will increase the percentage of FG fibers. In fact bodybuilders actually have a high percentage of SO fibers and very high muscle oxidative capacity (Tesch, Thorsson, Essen-Gustavsson 1989). Therefore, as the story goes, it helps if you can choose your parents for FG fibers as there is little you can do to increase the percentage of FG fibers you have, although with strength and power training you can increase the size of the FG fibers which makes them more capable to produce force and power. Along with the increase in FG fibers with strength and power training the FOG and SO fibers also increase in size and strength but to a somewhat lesser extent (Wilmore and Costill 1994).

CHANGES IN CAPILLARY DENSITY WITH AEROBIC TRAINING

Capillaries are the small vessels in between arterioles and venules (i.e., in between the arterial side of the body and venous side of the body). Capillaries are the blood delivery apparatus of the circulatory system. They deliver blood and remove metabolic by-products from the muscle. With training, the number of capillaries per muscle fiber goes up. Clearly, this is a good thing from both a metabolic by-product removal perspective and from a nutrient and oxygen delivery perspective. This means that the greater number of capillaries the greater perfusion of the muscle tissue in question. This results in better oxygen and nutrient delivery and the removal of hydrogen ions and lactic acid. This means that from the middle of the muscle fiber to the capillaries, the distance is decreased which allows for oxygen and nutrient delivery and the removal of metabolic by-products, to occur faster. This is a good thing for a wrestler as this means his physiology has improved. Interestingly, strength training with heavy weights without any other type of training will actually decrease capillary density relative to muscle fiber size as the distance from capillary to the middle of the muscle cell will become greater. This makes it more difficult to deliver oxygen-rich blood and nutrients (glucose, fatty acids, amino acids) and remove metabolic waste products (hydrogen ions and lactic acid) (Hudlicka 2011).

CHANGES IN MITOCHONDRIAL NUMBER AND FUNCTION

The mitochondria are called "the powerhouse of the cell", and they provide ATP or the energy currency of the cell at a much greater amount than conversion of glucose to lactic acid. You get 36–38 ATP for one glucose molecule with aerobic metabolism utilizing the mitochondria and 2–3 ATP utilizing glucose and going to lactic acid. Therefore, it is important to aerobically train and increase the number and function of your mitochondria so that you get a more oxidative fiber and greater yield of energy (Ingjer 1979).

CHANGES IN OXIDATIVE ENZYMES

Oxidative enzymes, many of which are contained in the middle of the mitochondria, increase with aerobic exercise training. These oxidative enzymes form energy exchange reactions with one another and capture the energy from glucose and fatty acids and possibly amino acids and make ATP. Again, you obtain much more energy (ATP) from combusting glucose oxidatively (using oxygen; 36–38 ATP) than breaking it down, anaerobically to lactic acid, also known as lactate (2–3 ATP). Additionally, during recovery from intense contractions such as during a wrestling match, the oxidative enzymes hasten recovery by allowing the resynthesis of ATP and phosphocreatine that were degraded by the intense exercise.

CHANGES IN LACTATE (LACTIC ACID) OXIDATION AND REMOVAL

About 75% of the lactic acid produced during exercise is combusted or oxidized for energy. Two concepts underlie this phenomenon. The intracellular lactate shuttle and the cell–cell lactate shuttle. In the intracellular lactate shuttle concept, lactate from muscle fibers is produced and oxidized in those same muscle fiber. In the cell–cell lactate shuttle lactate is produced in fast twitch glycolytic fibers and goes to slow twitch oxidative fibers for oxidation either by going to adjacent muscle fibers or circulating through the blood (Brooks, Fahey, and Baldwin 2005). Another fate of lactate is called the Cori Cycle, where lactate produced from muscle fibers goes to the liver through the blood stream and is converted to glucose. The glucose either gets converted to glycogen in the liver or goes back to the muscle and is used for fuel (Brooks, Fahey, and Baldwin 2005). These three mechanisms would appear to be important during wrestling as it is extremely intermittent with periods of intense lactic acid building time and periods of less intense exercise where lactate could be oxidized in the cell it was produced in, oxidized in an adjacent muscle fiber, or released into the circulation for conversion to glucose by the liver (Cori Cycle) (Table 8.2).

MUSCLE BUFFERING CAPACITY

The most important muscle buffering mechanism involved in buffering hydrogen ions is the presence of an amino acid derived substance carnosine (Harris et al. 2012; Harris and Stellingwerff 2013). Again, hydrogen ions can cause muscle fatigue by a number of mechanisms that involve energy metabolism and inhibition of muscle contraction (Green 2005). Furthermore, the vastus lateralis (thigh muscle) of bodybuilders has been shown to have the highest carnosine content ever recorded (Tallon et al 2005). This makes sense since when bodybuilders train they produce a lot of lactic acid. The increase in carnosine is likely an adaptation to the high muscle lactic acid concentrations. It follows that if one wants to increase the muscle carnosine concentrations to the greatest extent they should train like a bodybuilder, i.e., a high number of sets and repetitions. It is not uncommon for a bodybuilder to perform 20 sets for a given muscle group of 8–12 repetitions. See Lambert, Frank, and Evans (2004) for more information on bodybuilding training. This type of training could also be simulated by a high number of 30-second "Gos" during wrestling practices. Clearly, without barbells, wrestling, metabolically, is much like a 20 set per body

---

TABLE 8.2
Changes in Skeletal Muscle That Occur with Aerobic/Endurance Training

Fibers shift to a slower outward appearance and function

Mitochondrial number and function improve

Reduced lactic acid accumulation

Increase in oxidative enzymes

Increase in capillary density

Increase in myoglobin concentration

---

part bodybuilding workout with 30 seconds to 1 minute of rest between sets, and this is indicated by the high lactic acid levels in both wrestling (12.55 mmol/L for Elite wrestlers and 13.23 for Club-level wrestlers; Karnincic et al. 2009) and bodybuilding (Tesch, Thorsson, Essen-Gustavsson 1989) training.

KEY POINTS

1. Fast twitch fibers can become more slow in appearance and function with aerobic training.
2. Slow twitch fibers do not become more fast with anaerobic training.
3. Oxidative enzymes increase in muscle in response to aerobic training.
4. Mitochondrial number and function go up with aerobic exercise training.
5. Lactic acid accumulation in muscle and blood goes down with aerobic exercise training.
6. Capillary density increases in muscle with aerobic exercise training as does the muscle's oxygen carrying protein myoglobin.

9 Fuel Selection during a Wrestling Match

The major factor that dictates what fuel you use during exercise is the relative exercise intensity (% VO_2peak). The second factor that dictates which fuel you use during exercise is the training status of the athlete. The third factor that dictates fuel use is substrate availability. The greater the exercise intensity the greater the reliance on carbohydrate, while the lower the exercise intensity the greater the reliance on fat. The more highly endurance trained an individual is the greater the reliance on fat as a fuel up to higher intensities than in the untrained state. However, at intensities of exercise of ~80% VO_2peak, carbohydrate is still the predominant source of fuel for exercise even in the highly endurance trained individual (Brooks, Fahey, and Baldwin 2005). It is unlikely, under normal conditions, that exercise at 100% of VO_2 max is fueled by fat. However, McCartney et al. (1986) reported that fat contributed substantially to a fourth one-minute bout of high-intensity exercise with four minutes of rest between bouts. The caveat here is that power output declined substantially from bout 1 to bout 4, suggesting utilization of fat instead of carbohydrate will impair high-intensity exercise performance, and your best bet is to rely on carbohydrate for the performance of high-intensity exercise such as wrestling.

USE OF CARBOHYDRATE OR FAT DURING A WRESTLING MATCH

Fuel selection during exercise is largely dependent on the intensity of the exercise. Low-intensity activities burn fat and high-intensity activities burn carbohydrate. This is mainly because fat requires more oxygen to break down than carbohydrate. The reason for this is that carbohydrate has more oxygen in the molecule while fat has less oxygen in the fat molecule. Carbohydrates include carbon and water (of the denomination CH_2O) in different denominations while much of the fat less than the glycerol is made up of C–H (hydrocarbon) chains; therefore, more oxygen needs to be utilized, i.e., incorporated to break down a fat compared to carbohydrate. This is seen in the CO_2 produced relative to O_2 consumed for carbohydrate and fat (VCO_2 produced/VO_2 consumed; Respiratory Exchange Ratio; RER). It is a 1 to 1 ratio for pure carbohydrate and 0.7 for pure fat. That is you get much more CO_2 produced per given amount of oxygen for burning pure carbohydrate than for burning pure fat, i.e., you have to put less oxygen in for pure carbohydrate than pure fat. Burning fat is really a process that requires more time to do because you have to get oxygen in the lungs down the cellular level where fat oxidation can occur. For carbohydrates the oxygen is already in the molecule, and you don't have to put as much as oxygen in to get the CO_2 out. Carbohydrates can provide energy quickly, whereas fat takes longer to break down due to the oxygen requirements of fat breakdown. This can be changed somewhat by training (Brooks, Fahey, and White 2005) and keto-adapted diet (Burke et al. 2017). However, it would appear that the intensity of wrestling is too intense for substantial fat oxidation without about a 50% decline in force output (McCartney et al. 1986). This is not to say that fat cannot be used to restore energy (phosphocreatine and ATP) levels AFTER intense exercise. Data suggests that one minute very high-intensity bouts of exercise followed by four minutes of rest can result in a significant contribution by fat, especially the greater the number of bouts that are undertaken, i.e., fat utilization is greater after bout 4 than after bout 1 (McCartney et al 1986). However, power output went down dramatically over the course of one-minute bouts (McCartney et al. 1986). Additionally, Stellingwerf et al. (2006) and Constantin-Teodosiu et al. (2019) showed the enzyme used to oxidize carbohydrate during intense exercise (pyruvate dehydrogenase) is suppressed as a result of a high-fat diet. This means that less pyruvate is going to be converted to acetyl Co-A and enter the Krebs Cycle, leading to less ATP production and energy for muscle contraction. This clearly is a negative adaptation since carbohydrate provides ATP much more rapidly than fat. This is called greater metabolic power. Also, Burke et al. (2017) have shown that keto-adapted individuals burn more calories *during exercise* than their non-keto adapted counterparts suggesting less mechanical efficiency. This is in contrast to the effects of different types of diets on weight loss over the long haul (months), which seems to be regulated by energy balance (caloric balance) rather than whether someone is keto-adapted or not. Aragon et al. (2017) have concluded that the likely the best diets for weight loss and maintenance of muscle mass are high in protein and include weight training. Clearly, carbohydrates are the most important macronutrient for high-intensity exercise performance, and performance will suffer without adequate carbohydrates in the diet (Fleming et al. 2003; Langfort et al. 1997; Greenhaff et al. 1988a, 1988b; Ball, Greenhaff, and Maughan 1996; Maughan and Poole 1981; Maughan et al. 1997; Gleeson, Greenhaff, and Maughan 1988). These are two separate situations: optimal weight loss and optimal performance, which should be treated separately (Lambert and Jones 2010).

In a classic set of experiments starting in 1981 Maughan's group had preempted the Keto craze and put a spear through the heart of it. In the first study, Maughan and Poole (1981) had subjects exercise to exhaustion at 104% VO$_2$max. This was done on three occasions. First after exhaustive prolonged exercise followed by three days of a normal carbohydrate diet, then after exhaustive exercise followed by a low carbohydrate diet, and then after exhaustive exercise followed by a high-carbohydrate diet. Exercise time to exhaustion at 104% VO$_2$max was reduced by 32% from normal diet to low diet, increased by 36% from a high-carbohydrate diet to a normal carbohydrate diet, and improved by 100% comparing a high-carbohydrate diet to a low carbohydrate diet. The key to this study was that each exercise test to exhaustion was preceded by an exhaustive exercise. Thus, they evaluated different diets when "exercise training" was being undertaken. In a subsequent study, Greenhaff, Gleeson, and Maughan (1988a) evaluated 4 days of dietary manipulation without "exercise training" on time to exhaustion at 100% VO$_2$max. They found that a high-fat high-protein diet reduced performance by 14.8% from a Normal diet. A similar reduction in performance was observed when comparing a high-fat high-protein diet to a high-carbohydrate diet. The difference in the magnitude of the impairment of performance between Maughan and Poole's study (1981) and Greenhaff, Gleeson, and

Maughan's study (1988a) was the fact that the diets were preceded by "exhaustive exercise" prior to the diet and subsequent exercise test at 100% VO_2max to exhaustion. In a third study, Greenhaff, Gleeson, and Maughan (1988b) used standardized high-intensity exercise of 3 minutes duration and undertook a diet without prior exercise on muscle metabolism and acid–base status. They found that muscle glycogen was augmented by 23% on the high-carbohydrate diet. Additionally, they found that muscle pH declined 104% greater on the high-fat high-protein diet than the high-carbohydrate diet. Thus, two things go on: muscle pH is negatively affected by a high-fat high-protein diet and when you couple this with "exhaustive exercise", there is reduced availability of muscle glycogen and a much greater reduction in exercise performance than when the diets were not preceded by "exhaustive exercise". The carbohydrate dependence of exercise also appears to be the case during low-intensity long-duration exercise (i.e., race walking; Burke et al. 2017), although calorie burning during exercise is better on a ketogenic diet than on a high-carbohydrate diet; thereby, performance is impaired likely because of the greater oxygen cost of exercise, i.e., less mechanical efficiency.

KEY POINTS

1. Fuel selection during exercise is dependent primarily on exercise intensity and substrate availability.
2. Research has shown in "untrained individuals" that at the intensity a wrestling match is conducted at, 100% of energy needs is supplied by carbohydrate with 99% coming from muscle glycogen and 1% coming from blood glucose.
3. When "high-intensity exercise" is undertaken, such as in a wrestling match, with low muscle glycogen stores, fat can assist in energy provision, but the power output declines drastically.
4. Training can improve the reliance on the aerobic utilization of glucose and ATP yield, but the extent of this increased reliance on blood glucose appears to be limited during very high-intensity exercise.

10 Energy Systems and Biochemical Causes of Fatigue

The first source of energy during intense muscle contraction is stored ATP and Phosphocreatine (PCr). This lasts from about 10 to 30 seconds depending on the intensity of exercise. Within seconds of the commencement of exercise muscle glycogen starts to break down. The production of lactic acid from this process produces 3 ATP from each glucose derived from glycogen. A consequence, however, of this glycogen breakdown is lactic acid accumulation in muscle. The hydrogen ion (H^+) associated with the lactic acid production can cause muscular fatigue. The cause of fatigue between 30 and 90 seconds is likely acidosis. This acidosis can cause a number of problems with muscle contraction and energy metabolism (McComas 1996). The next way that glycogen is broken down is by aerobic means. The aerobic breakdown of muscle glycogen yields 39 ATP per glucose derived from muscle glycogen. This tends to happen after about 60–90 seconds of high-intensity exercise. Other potential fuels at this time appear to intramuscular lipid. However, we are not sure if this substrate is used or just lysed and liberated into the blood stream. Likely, during intermittent exercise at 95%–100% of VO_2max, such as amateur wrestling, the fuel sources for exercise are confined to ATP-PCr and the anaerobic and aerobic use of muscle glycogen. This may slightly change to blood glucose in trained individuals but clearly not much blood glucose is oxidized at 100% of VO_2max as only 1% of the energy derived for exercise at 97% of VO_2max was blood glucose with remaining 99% coming from muscle glycogen in untrained individuals (Katz et al. 1986). Also, you will use more fat in the glycogen depleted state but a side effect of this increased fat utilization is that performance suffers (McCartney et al. 1986).

Within the skeletal muscle are two energy stores, such as ATP and PCr (ATP-PC). The onset of use of these energy stores is immediate and lasts for at the most 30 seconds (Brooks, Fahey, and Baldwin 2005). If exercise intensity surpasses the stores within this system, force generating capacity will be impaired in as little as 30 seconds. Also, within the skeletal muscle are stores of muscle carbohydrate called muscle glycogen. Muscle glycogen degradation to lactic acid can happen in as few as 10 seconds (Jacobs et al. 1983). Within 90 seconds lactic acid and its associated protons (H^+) can build up and inhibit muscle contraction (Green 2005). For exercise lasting longer than 90 seconds aerobic oxidation of muscle glycogen and blood glucose predominate. The level of muscle glycogen and blood glucose will dictate how long a person can exercise relying on these fuels. During prolonged exercise at 75% of VO_2max a low-carbohydrate diet will lead to exhaustion in about 60 minutes, a normal carbohydrate diet will result in exhaustion in about 100 minutes, and a high-carbohydrate diet for 3 days will result in exhaustion in about 190 minutes (Bergstrom et al. 1967). This is about a ~215% improvement in time to exhaustion during moderate-intensity exercise. At this intensity of exercise there is considerable fat oxidation. In a sport like wrestling the carbohydrate dependence and fat oxidation are less due to the intensity of exercise being near 100% VO$_2$max. Amateur wrestling is conducted at an intensity of ~95%–100% of VO$_2$max. Therefore, a wrestler needs to make sure he has adequate carbohydrate available for exercise of this intensity. Additionally, as many as five matches can be wrestled in a day (Lambert and Jones 2010). If adequate carbohydrate stores are not attained prior to that day, fatigue can ensue due to carbohydrate depletion of active muscle (Tables 10.1 and 10.2).

TABLE 10.1

Energy Sources for Exercise, Requirement for Oxygen, and the Order with Which they Are Used During Exercise at 90%–100% of VO$_2$max

Source	Requirement for Oxygen	Order of Utilization
ATP-PCr	Anaerobic	First (Clearly used during a 6–7-minute match)
Muscle glycogen	Anaerobic	Second (Clearly used during a 6–7-minute match)
Muscle glycogen	Aerobic	Third (Clearly used during a 6–7-minute match). Training augments the aerobic use of carbohydrate at high intensities of exercise
Blood glucose	Aerobic can be used to resynthesize muscle glycogen during intermittent anaerobic exercise	Fourth (Provides only 1% of used carbohydrate during exercise at 97% of VO$_2$max in untrained subjects; Katz et al. (1986)
(Intramuscular lipid)	(Aerobic; however, we are not sure whether they are utilized or just undergo breakdown as a result of exercise. These stores are dependent on training status rather than diet)	(Likely in a tie for third)

TABLE 10.2

Duration of Exercise and Potential Causes of Fatigue

Duration of Maximal Continuous Dynamic Exercise	Potential Causes of Fatigue
0–30 seconds	ATP and PC depletion
30–90 seconds	Lactic acid accumulation
90 seconds to 1.5 hours	Unknown, could be low muscle glycogen if glycogen is low to begin with, could be acidosis from lactic acid accumulation, hypohydration if fluid is not replaced
1.5–3.0 hours	Most evidence points to muscle glycogen depletion although hypohydration would play a role if fluid is not replaced

KEY POINTS

1. Depending on the intensity of exercise the ATP and PCr stores can be depleted in as little as a few seconds or may be able to last for about 30 seconds. Thus, if the intensity of wrestling is high, fatigue could ensue rather quickly due to the depletion of these two substrates.
2. Hydrogen ion accumulation from lactic acid production can cause fatigue at a number of sites on the contractile apparatus and energy metabolism and is thought to cause fatigue in high-intensity exercise lasting 30–90 seconds.
3. For events lasting 90 seconds to 1.5 hours it is believed that reduced muscle glycogen stores could be the possible cause of fatigue. Thus, reduced muscle glycogen is a probable cause of fatigue during a wrestling match and the more matches you wrestle, the greater the potential for this to be the case.
4. For events lasting 1.5–3 hours the cause of fatigue is less well known but likely is reduced muscle glycogen and/or reduced hydration levels if fluid is not ingested.

11 Physiological Factors That Allow for the Attainment of "Maximal Power Output" and "Entire Match Wrestling Power Output"

"Maximal Power Output" is mainly dependent on Force output. Getting strong (high force output) will also make you faster (time component of the Power equation). Thus, to develop "Maximal Power Output", one of the factors I have identified as important to wrestling success, you need to get stronger. The other component I have identified as important to wrestling success is "Entire Match Wrestling Power Output". This is dependent on maximal force, anaerobic capacity, and critical power. Maximal force also greatly affects anaerobic capacity, as measured by the Wingate Test and the Maximal Accumulated Oxygen Deficit. Thus, for "Entire Match Wrestling Power Output" you need to get strong. Also, longer "go's" (1–3 minutes) will develop muscle buffering capacity and therefore anaerobic capacity. The last component "Critical Power" is the maximal power output that can be maintained that is purely fueled by aerobic metabolism. This component can be trained by 5–10 minutes intervals at 80%–90% of VO_2max and long slow-distance training.

"Maximal Power Output" would be defined as Force × (Distance/Time). The distance you move a weight during weight training, for example, does not change. However, Force can change and the Time it takes to generate the force can change. We generally think of Force as Maximal Strength or in weight lifting terms the One Repetition Maximum. So maximal power output is dictated by how much strength you generate in fastest amount of time possible. Maximal Force Generating capacity is thought to be determined by a number of factors. Much of this maximal force generating capacity is due to the nervous system. Some of it is due to muscle fiber type which you really can't change to a faster fiber and muscle fiber size which you can change dramatically. One such neurological phenomenon is Motor Unit Recruitment. That is how many nerves and the fibers connected to them can you incorporate into a movement. Generally speaking, when motor unit recruitment is greater, the greater the level of voluntary effort expressed, and can be trained via things like strength and power training. Another neurological factor is motor unit firing rates, and this occurs as a result of a greater impulse "volley" down a motor neuron to all of the muscle fibers it connects to. The greater the number of impulses down a motor neuron, the greater the force production of that motor unit (all the muscle fibers attached to that motor neuron). With regard to fiber type, the more fast myosin a muscle fiber has, the faster it will contract at a given force adding to "Maximal Muscle Power", since this takes into account maximal force and the speed at which it is generated. Additionally, the larger the muscle fiber, regardless of how much fast myosin it has, the greater its force generating capacity. What is less clear from traditional literature is if you train a muscle at faster speeds with lower loads (as you have to do as Force and Velocity are somewhat inversely proportional), if it will become faster and therefore augment the Distance/Time component of the Power calculation = Force × (Distance/Time). The maximal power output of a muscle is at one-third of maximal force output or at a force equivalent to one-third of maximal shortening velocity. It is unclear whether training at one-third of maximal force output at fast speeds will produce better power output than training with high loads (Enoka 2008) at the present time. However, we do know that the stimulus is different but may not be any better than training with high loads. Also, we know training with light loads at maximal speeds may increase the risk of injury. So, at present this author's suggestion is not to train with light loads at maximal speeds due to the risk of injury (Behm and Sale 1993). Many times in amateur wrestling this is moot point as isometric or slow muscle contractions are utilized. However, fast contractions are also utilized: for example a wrestler shooting in on a high crotch takedown as fast as he can to get there before the defending wrestler can turn the corner. In this case it is body weight (say 149 lbs) as the force and a time factor determined by how quickly the athlete can get to the leg (Table 11.1).

Question: Is there a place for high-speed contractions to develop power?

The research suggests that high force contractions are much more important at developing power than high-speed contractions. However, the research is lacking in the number of studies done with large muscle groups and multiple joint contractions. It is possible and probable that high-speed contractions increase the concentration of proteins *inherent to skeletal muscle integrity* (Trappe et al. 2002). High-speed contractions like eccentric contractions can induce significant skeletal muscle soreness and likely damage. It is also possible that the connective tissues within skeletal muscle such as endomysium, perimysium, and epimysium adapt to these

---

TABLE 11.1
Neurological and Fiber Muscle Type Characteristics That Determine Maximal Force Generating Capacity

Motor unit recruitment
Motor unit firing rates
Muscle fiber type
Muscle fiber size

---

high-speed contractions. Therefore, the athletes and coaches may be ahead of the researchers. If you can avoid injury, high-speed contractions likely are beneficial for improving athletic performance, i.e., improving power.

IMPROVING "ENTIRE MATCH WRESTLING POWER OUTPUT"

To improve "Entire Match Wrestling Power Output", one must be strong or stronger. That is, have high force generating capacity. Interestingly, in a study we published in 2013 (Lambert et al. 2013) comparing time to fatigue between men and women at 100% of VO_2peak, the men went 48% longer than the women. However, when we expressed the time to fatigue relative to the amount of fat-free mass (a surrogate for muscle mass) they had, there were no differences between the men and the women. What this means is that muscle mass or more correctly muscle strength was likely the reason for the much longer time to fatigue for men than women. The time to fatigue for the men was roughly 4.5 minutes and for the women 3 minutes. What this indicates is that maximal force generating capacity is a great indicator of your ability to stave off short-term exercise fatigue. Thus, this would indicate if you want to get less fatigable for wrestling, get stronger!

Another key factor thought to assist with staving off fatigue is the muscle carnosine content which is a muscle buffer. Interestingly, Roger Harris's group (Tallon et al. 2005) has found that muscle carnosine is highest in bodybuilders who perform many sets of weight lifting exercises for a given muscle group. So to reduce your fatigability train heavy and with many sets. This could also be simulated on a wrestling mat with 30 maximal "Go's" at an intensity greater than normal for a full 6–7-minute match.

Another way to improve "Entire Match Wrestling Power Output" is to improve "Critical Power" which is the maximal sustainable intensity at which aerobic metabolism provides all of the energy needs for exercise. A way to do this is to improve aerobic metabolism via long-duration (10 minutes) intervals or long slow-distance training.

KEY POINTS

1. To improve "Maximal Power Output" the primary means should be to improve maximal force generating capacity or "strength". It is possible that "speed training" is useful but limited research data is available on this prospect.
2. To improve "Entire Match Power Output" again you need to improve "strength" as this will prolong your time to fatigue. Additionally, improving muscle buffering capacity by training with multiple 30 "Go's" would seem to be an excellent way to improve muscle buffering capacity.
3. An additional way to improve "Entire Match Wrestling Power Output" is to improve "Critical Power" which is the sustainable intensity at which aerobic metabolism is at a maximum.

12 Cardiovascular Adaptations to Endurance Exercise

Endurance training whether continuous or intermittent in nature will increase how much blood the heart pumps per minute: Cardiac Output, mainly by increasing maximal stroke volume (blood pumped per beat) with no change in Heart Rate (beats per minute). The size of the left ventricle of the heart is also enlarged with endurance training. Blood volume or specifically plasma volume is a determinant of stroke volume as the greater the plasma volume the greater the venous return and the more blood the heart will pump. Blood volume increases with training. Cardiac output is one of the major determinants of VO_2max/peak which is also dictated by the Arteriovenous Oxygen Difference (A-VO_2diff) which means extraction of oxygen at the tissue level: VO_2max/peak = CO × A-VO_2diff. A-VO_2diff is improved by an increase in capillarity in muscle beds, mitochondrial number and function, and mitochondrial enzymes.

Stroke volume is the maximal amount of blood the heart can pump per beat. Heart rate is the number of times the heart beats per minute. Cardiac Output is the product of Heart rate and Stroke volume (CO = HR × SV). Maximal heart rate (the maximal rate attained during maximal exercise) does not increase as a result of endurance training but submaximal heart rate goes down as a result of training. This is due to the increase in plasma volume as a result of an increase in plasma albumin that accompanies endurance exercise training (Wilmore and Costill 1994). This has implications for performance as protein malnutrition will result in a low plasma albumin concentration, and thus a reduced plasma volume in turn will reduce stroke volume, cardiac output, and VO_2 max. This clearly would be deleterious to wrestling performance as wrestling is performed at about 100% of VO_2 max. If protein is too low or energy is too low in the diet, albumin may drop reducing VO_2max. Maximal Stroke volume increases as a result of endurance exercise training, and this results in an increase in cardiac output despite no increase in maximal heart rate. VO_2 max is the product of the cardiac output (Stroke volume × Heart Rate) and the ability of the muscles to extract oxygen from the blood called A-VO_2 difference (CO × A-VO_2diff = VO_2). VO_2max, the single best predictor of a person's fitness level obviously, goes up with endurance training. Evidence that dehydration will undermine your training adaptations is brought about by the fact that dehydration lowers plasma volume. This would occur by losing fluids through sweating which lowers plasma volume. A lowered plasma volume will result in a lowered max stroke volume which will lower cardiac output and VO_2max. Since wrestlers exercise at close to VO_2max (95%–100%; Gleeson et al. 1988; Lambert and Jones 2010) this will result in lowering of your performance on the mat. That is dehydration will impair your maximal fitness level, and wrestling is dependent on your maximal fitness levels (Tables 12.1 and 12.2).

TABLE 12.1
Cardiovascular Adaptations to Endurance Training

Increase in cardiac output
Increase in stroke volume
No change in max heart rate; reduction in resting heart rate
Increase in A-VO$_2$diff
Increase in plasma volume
Increase in venous return during exercise
Increase in left ventricular heart muscle mass
Increase in the number and size of the mitochondria
Increase in the number of capillaries perfusing muscle

TABLE 12.2
Effects of Dehydration on Cardiovascular Variables

Heart rate	Increases
Stroke volume	Decreases
Cardiac output	Decreases
A-VO$_2$ difference	No change

KEY POINTS

1. The cardiovascular system adapts to exercise training by increasing the ability of the heart to pump blood and improving the ability of the tissues to take up oxygen due to increased capillarity.
2. The heart will adapt to exercise by pumping more blood per beat of the heart (i.e., increased Stroke Volume). This is due to a greater plasma volume; the heart pumps what is returned to it and greater muscularity of the left ventricle.
3. There is no change in maximal heart rate with training but resting heart rate goes down due to improved venous return.
4. Dehydration reduces plasma volume and venous return to the heart and cardiac output while increasing heart rate.
5. Protein or energy (kcals or kilojoules) malnutrition may lower blood albumin concentrations and would lower plasma volume and VO$_2$peak.

13 Training Variables

Training variables can be broken down into frequency, intensity, volume, and duration. Frequency is how often you train, intensity is the effort that you train at, volume is how much work performed, and duration is how long it takes. Training volume has received the most attention in the literature and it appears that training once per day is as effective as training twice per day with regard to physical conditioning and subsequent race times during competition in competitive swimmers. Those that trained twice per day over the course of their four-year collegiate career saw similar improvements as those that trained once per day. However, aside from swimming (which relies heavily on muscular endurance) which is assessed by race times, there is a good rationale for training twice per day in competitive amateur wrestlers. Strength acquisition and skill acquisition through drilling can be done in a second practice in competitive wrestlers while the primary practice deals with live wrestling. Another reason for training twice per day would be to obtain additional aerobic training during the second practice. However, the Coach and Athlete must be cognizant of overtraining while training twice per day and should monitor variables that would be indicative of overtraining (see "Physiological Assessment and Determination of Overtraining" chapter).

FREQUENCY

Means how often you train.

INTENSITY

Means how hard you train. This is often expressed as the percentage of VO_2max, percentage of heart rate max, or in terms of the rating of perceived exertion (Borg 1982).

VOLUME/DURATION

This in terms of wrestling means time spent wrestling at a given intensity. With regard to running, it means distance covered, etc.

TRAINING VOLUME

The question of how much to train at a given intensity is an important and elusive question. Data from swimmers suggest training 4–6 hours/day, 5–6 days/week is no better than training 1–1.5 hours/day (Costill et al. 1991) with regard to short-term endurance performance and may actually hinder strength and sprint performance.

TABLE 13.1

Training Variables for a Given Type of Exercise

Frequency

Intensity

Volume and duration

Additionally, those swimmers who swam greater than 10,000 m/day (4–6 hours/day) over the course of their 4-year collegiate career saw a 0.8% improvement in performance in the 100 m front crawl event (primarily anaerobic) which was the same as the 0.8% improvement over the 4-year career for swimmers who swam less than 5,000 m/day (1–1.5 hours/day) (Costill and Wilmore 1994). Thus, excessive training volume is not the answer and may actually lead to poorer performances during competition than low–moderate volumes of training. Given the probability of glycogen depletion and overtraining or overtraining without glycogen depletion, excessive training is not the answer (Table 13.1).

TO TRAIN ONCE OR TWICE PER DAY FOR WRESTLING?

With regard to one a day or two a day practices for wrestling, the answer is it depends. Training intensely with only live wrestling for 4 hours/day is not the answer as you will probably have the same lack of improvement over long periods of time as the swimmers in the preceding example (i.e., study of Costill et al. 1991). However, for example, if you have different goals for different practices, i.e., strength training in the morning and live wrestling in the evening one day, drilling in the morning and live wrestling (100% effort) in evening on another day, this would be feasible from a chronic fatigue standpoint. Clearly, two practices per day where they are all live wrestling is not conducive to positive adaptations in performance similar to the lack of results the swimmers in the preceding study saw. That being said, for collegiate wrestlers and above, two a day practices may be the way to go because of their increased daily flexibility due to class schedules and the fact this keeps them on task. Also, new skill acquisition and motor learning through drilling new technique take considerable time and two a day practices are conducive to this. As seen in the research example above from swimmers, they may peak in their physiological potential (i.e., the 0.8% improvement for both groups over four years suggest little room for improvement after high school) before they get to college also by engaging in two a day practices. Again it should be noted that two a day practices that are not the same, i.e., live wrestling in both practices are likely beneficial to the student-athlete for reasons other than increased training volume (i.e., skill acquisition, strength development, fat burning aerobic exercise, and long slow distance). A training session should consist of a warm-up, conditioning, cool down, and stretching and should be specific for the physical attribute desired. That is the workout should follow the principle of Specific Adaptations to Imposed Demands (Table 13.2).

TABLE 13.2
Pros and Cons of Training Twice per Day

Pros	Cons
Allows adequate time for skill acquisition during a second practice	Requires double the time for athletes and coaches
Allows adequate time for resistance training during a second practice	Clearly, requires as much if not more supervision at the high-school level and lower than actual practice
Allows adequate time for "extra" aerobic conditioning, i.e., a long run	If markers of overtraining/training stress are not monitored it could lead to overtraining
The extra dedication is likely advantageous as high-intensity training is effective	The training, if not matched by equal energy (calories), carbohydrate, and protein intake to that utilized during training could lead to Relative Energy Deficiency in Sport. Additionally, if sleep and rest are inadequate overtraining syndrome could occur

COMPONENTS OF A TRAINING SESSION (I.E., STRUCTURE OF A PRACTICE)

A training session should consist of a warm-up, conditioning, cool down, and stretching (ACSM 2014).

WARM-UP AND FLEXIBILITY

Clearly, warm-up and flexibility training are important parts of any wrestling training session. It is commonly accepted that warm-up (consisting of both passive warming and active warm-up) reduces the risk of injury and improves exercise performance (Knudson 2008) by increased blood flow and oxygen delivery to the muscle. Passive warming could be something like a heating pad, whirlpool, or hot shower prior to the training session. Active warm-up consists of light calisthenics for 5–10 minutes followed by wrestling-specific low-intensity aerobic activities for 5–10 minutes (ACSM 2014). Flexibility training is important from the standpoint of improving the range of motion of a joint and performance but not for injury prevention (Knudson 2008). Flexibility training should be performed AFTER the training session during the cool-down period. There are three reasons for this: (1) A warm tissue is less likely to be injured (Knudson 2008), (2) It does not matter where in the workout flexibility training is as far as improvements in flexibility, (3) It is commonly known that there can be exercise performance impairment following stretching. According to Knudson (2008), flexibility training should be at least three times per week after moderate to vigorous physical activity, and the muscle should be held with a low level of force after being slowly elongated, 4–5 stretches (total body) should be held for 15–30 seconds, and stretches should be conducted either in a static manner (no movement at the point of the stretch) or using proprioceptive neuromuscular facilitation (contract the muscle with no change in muscle length followed by a relaxation and stretch; Knudson 2008).

CONDITIONING

The next few sections will deal with conditioning portion of each training session, which includes all forms of wrestling, running, calisthenics, and resistance training.

PROPER AROUSAL LEVELS FOR SKILL PERFORMANCE AND CONDITIONING

Based on our knowledge of motor learning (Magill 1985), to perform a skill optimally, you need the right level of arousal. For complicated skills this follows an inverted-U theory and for non-complicated skills they follow the Drive Theory. The inverted-U theory states that a medium level of arousal is required for optimal performance of a complicated skill such as throwing a football accurately. The Drive Theory states that for uncomplicated skills such as the deadlift, the greater the arousal the better the performance on the skill. These are important because if you have high arousal levels with a complicated skill you will make mistakes. Low arousal with an uncomplicated skill and you will have suboptimal performance, for example, only being able to deadlift 135 lbs instead of 185 lbs. For wrestling I believe about a 50%–75% arousal level (subjectively determined) may be appropriate as the great strength and power requirements of wrestling require arousal while the high-technique requirement dictates less than maximal arousal levels. This would be about 50–75% of the arousal level you would want if doing a one repetition maximum deadlift. However, my contention should be followed up with research.

SAID PRINCIPLE: SPECIFIC ADAPTATIONS TO IMPOSED DEMANDS

This means you obtain the adaptations you train for. If you want to train for anaerobic adaptations train in bouts less than 2–3 minutes (primary energy sources anaerobic; ATP-PCr and lactic acid). If you want to train for aerobic adaptations train for durations longer than 2–3 minutes. However, there is crossover. For example, training with aerobic intervals you stress both anaerobic and aerobic systems. Additionally, training with anaerobic intervals, for example, one minute intervals with four minutes of rest you will stress both anaerobic and aerobic systems. Again, you obtain the adaptations you train for but there is crossover between the adaptations of the anaerobic and aerobic energy systems and therefore the type of adaptations you obtain.

DURATION OF A CONDITIONING SESSION

This most likely should be based on the nutritional status of student-athletes. What I am talking about here is the carbohydrate intake of the wrestlers. If the wrestler is taking in less than 4 g CHO (carbohydrate)/kilogram body weight, intense conditioning should be less than one hour. If the carbohydrate intake is between

4 and 6 g CHO/kilogram body weight the intense conditioning portion of the practice should be about one hour. If the wrestler is taking in 8–10 g CHO/kilogram body weight intense conditioning can be longer than 1.5–2 hours. Why is this? Because carbohydrate is limiting to intense exercise performance. When you use up all the carbohydrate in muscle, blood, and liver the athlete will become hypoglycemic. Endurance athletes call this "bonking". Clearly, you cannot perform measurable exercise while hypoglycemic and it is downright dangerous. At the intensity of exercise that wrestlers compete at (95%–100% VO_2max) carbohydrate provides equal to or greater (by my estimation based on Katz et al. (1986); 100% carbohydrate used at 97% of VO_2max in an untrained person and assuming a highly trained athlete) than 95% of fuel necessary for completion of the match. Thus, carbohydrate status should dictate the volume of intense conditioning the wrestler does, i.e., duration of live wrestling during practice.

COOL DOWN

A cool down should consist of ~5–10 minutes of low to moderate (20%–50% of VO_2max) cardiovascular as well as muscular endurance activities (ACSM 2014).

KEY POINTS

1. The variables for training can be broken down into Intensity, Frequency, and Volume/Duration.
2. Training twice a day is warranted if the overall intensity (% of VO_2max) of one of the sessions is substantially lower (i.e., skill acquisition; drilling) than the other session which should be of high intensity.
3. The duration of the conditioning session during wrestling exercise should be dictated by the nutritional status (i.e., carbohydrate status) of the athletes.
4. The components of a training session should consist of warm-up, the conditioning session, and cool down.

14 Training

One factor, in particular, determines your "Maximal Power Output" and that is "Maximal Force" (Strength). Three factors appear to dictate your "Entire Match Wrestling Power Output": (1) Maximal Force Output, (2) Anaerobic Capacity, and (3) Critical Power.

"Maximal Force Output" has a profound effect on your ability to generate power for the whole 6–7 minutes. Typically, you train for "Maximal Force Output" with strength training. Anaerobic Capacity is the maximal ability to generate energy anaerobically by the working muscles. Much of Anaerobic Capacity is determined by Maximal Force Output (Medbo et al. 1988; Medbo and Tabata 1993; Lambert et al. 2013). Also, training with 30-second to 1-minute maximal intervals and 2–3 minutes intervals at about 100% of VO_2peak will also improve your Anaerobic Capacity. Critical Power is the maximal power output where the energy provision is solely aerobic (Poole et al. 2016). This component can be trained by performing high-intensity but aerobic intervals of 5–10 minutes in duration, which has been shown to produce an almost immediate and profound increase in mitochondrial number and density in young healthy subjects (Spina et al. 1996). I will expand on these training principles in subsequent sections (Table 14.1).

TRAINING FOR OPTIMAL STRENGTH (FORCE)

Having improved strength is advantageous for wrestlers. Having strength for strengths' sake (for example, pulling in a double leg takedown, lifting, throws, riding, or getting out from the bottom using a stand-up), and also for improved 4–7 minute high-intensity exercise capacity (Lambert et al. 2013) as strength dictates time to fatigue at this exercise duration, is important for wrestlers of all ages. According to Kraemer and Fleck (1993) strength training can start as young as 7 years of age with emphasis on technique and no progressive overload, except for bodyweight utilized calisthenics. As age progresses, more emphasis can be placed on progressive

---

TABLE 14.1

Influence of Maximal Force Output (Strength with Accompanying Muscle Mass) on Physiology

Increases muscle power (Behm and Sale 1993)

Increases time to fatigue (Lambert et al. 2013)

Increases anaerobic capacity (Medbo et al. 1988; Medbo and Tabata 1993) increases VO_2peak (Lambert et al. 2020)

Theoretically increases arteriovenous oxygen difference (Lambert 2019)

Theoretically increases venous return (Lambert 2019)

Theoretically increases stroke volume (Lambert 2019)

---

overload with a continued emphasis on technique. When the child reaches the age of 16 he or she can begin using adult types of resistance training (Kraemer and Fleck 1993).

PRINCIPLES FOR OFF-SEASON STRENGTH TRAINING AND SAMPLE STRENGTH TRAINING WORKOUTS

A beginning weight trainer will get strong on any workout because it is a novel stimulus to the neuromuscular system (Sale 1988). In fact, the greatest strength gains are made in the first 6 months of a strength training regimen (Sale 1988). As you continue on a strength training regimen after gaining considerable strength there will be a leveling off in strength gains. The idea at this point is *change* strength training regimens, so you can continue gaining strength and reach a new strength training plateau (Figure 14.1). The first workout that should be undertaken is 1 set of 10 repetitions for 6 movements aimed at the legs, back, chest, shoulders, triceps, and biceps. This should be performed three times per week. After, plateaus in strength following this regimen add two sets to each exercise. This is called the Delorme method (Delorme and Watkins 1948; 3 sets × 10 reps). Somewhere in your training history, when a plateau is reached you need to switch to each body part getting trained two times per week. This added recovery is required as you progress and gets stronger and adds sets to your workout. As the higher intensity (percentage of one repetition maximum) workouts will require a longer recovery period for progress (my experience after 38–39 years of resistance training; and by experience, this is how Powerlifters train). The reason for this is unknown but could involve the central nervous system and/or stress hormone secretion (epinephrine and cortisol) as muscle soreness actually gets less the more trained you are. Another explanation is subclinical muscle inflammation (i.e., no soreness but impaired function) as a result of higher force outputs. I would suggest shifting to a four day a week routine where

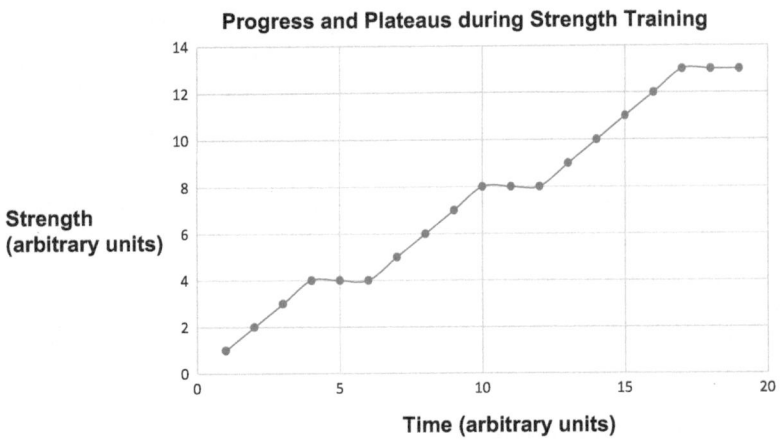

FIGURE 14.1 Progress and plateaus during strength training.

TABLE 14.2

Off-Season *Strength* Training Guidelines

	Beginner	Intermediate	Advanced
Sets	1–3 × 6 exercises Whole body each workout	4 × 12 exercises Half the body each workout	4 × 12 exercises One or two muscle groups per workout
Reps	10	4–6	1–4
Days/week for a muscle group	3	2	1
Days/week total	3	4	1–5

each muscle group is trained twice per week. Ultimately, for maximal strength gains you should probably only train each muscle group heavy one time per week. This is what elite Powerlifters do because of the extreme taxing effects that occur from their high-intensity (high percentage of 1 repetition maximum (RM)) workouts. The underlying mechanism for the prolonged recovery as you advance in strength gains you switch to lower repetition workouts something like 4 sets of 4 repetitions for each exercise at the same weight is unknown. Other advanced workouts for strength are performing 5, 4, 3, 2, and 1 repetitions with increasing weight and the one repetition lift being about 90% of your one repetition maximum (the greatest weight you can lift one time). This is an area of Exercise Physiology research where guidelines can be proposed but nothing is set in stone. Additionally, do not compare yourself to other individuals as your progress may be faster or slower than them in strength gains. The idea is to keep your weights moving up. As a guideline, leveling off of progress would be lack of a 5 lbs increase in two weeks of training. A 2.5 kg (5 lbs) increase every 2 weeks is a slow but steady progress. Please see Table 14.2 for a summary of Off-Season Strength Training.

IN-SEASON STRENGTH TRAINING

Generally speaking, the idea behind in-season strength training is that you should maintain the gains in strength you made in the off-season. This is no easy task with hard wrestling workouts and potentially suboptimal nutrition (See Lambert and Jones 2010). So it is likely that you should only train each muscle group once per week during the season. This is probably sufficient for strength maintenance during the season (Trappe, Costill, and Thomas et al. 2002).

Training for Optimal Strength usually involves sets of between 3 and 6 repetitions although Powerlifters and Olympic lifters typically perform repetitions as low as one repetition while getting ready for competition. The difficult part comes with determining how many sets and the optimal repetition regimen (i.e., 5 sets of 5, 3 sets of 3, 10 sets of 1, etc.). For a detailed summary of how to train for strength in children please see position stands by the American College of Sports Medicine and the National Strength and Conditioning Association.

TRAINING FOR MAXIMAL POWER

In contrast to contemporary thinking that you need to train fast to increase power (Force × Distance/Time), strength training (slow speeds) is a great way to train for power which encompasses both strength and the speed of movement (Force × Distance/Time). This was illustrated in a classic study by Behm and Sale (1993) in which the *intended* movement velocity was more important than the actual movement velocity for velocity specific training adaptations. What does this mean in the real world? *Train with heavy weights and intend or try to move them fast even though they may move slow.* This will develop strength at fast velocities (speeds) or power. Additionally, this approach may be safer than moving light weights at high velocities during training which could lead to joint and muscle injuries.

TRAINING FOR OPTIMAL ANAEROBIC CAPACITY

Anaerobic means without oxygen. The energy systems that contribute to anaerobic energy metabolism are the degradation of adenosine triphosphate (ATP) and Phosphocreatine (PCr) as well as glycogenolysis/glycolysis to lactic acid. Anaerobic Capacity is defined by performance on the "All Out" 30-second Wingate Anaerobic Exercise Test in which Peak Anaerobic Power, Mean Anaerobic Power, and a fatigue index can be determined. Clearly the Wingate test is a measure of ATP and PC stores, the capacity to produce energy through glycogenolysis, and glycolysis to lactic acid. Additionally, Peak Anaerobic Power is a measure of instantaneous muscle power. For anaerobic capacity, strength training (3–6 repetitions per set) will assist in the ATP-PC portion of the exercise (first 6 seconds) in which the Peak Anaerobic Power is usually generated. Power encompasses how fast the work can be done or work per unit time (Force × Distance/Time). Clearly 30-second to 1-minute intervals will improve anaerobic capacity. Children have lower levels of the key glycolytic enzyme phosphofructokinase (Wilmore and Costill 1994). Children, however, can adapt to anaerobic training with increases in phosphofructokinase and maximal lactate concentrations (Wilmore and Costill 1994). My gut opinion is that for young kids you should avoid things like Tabata intervals (Tabata et al. 1996; 20 seconds maximal, 10 seconds rest). Additionally, focusing on things like improving strength through strength training (kids age 7 and up; Kraemer and Fleck 1993) will increase neuromuscular components and likely increase anaerobic exercise capacity (Lambert and Jones 2010) as fat-free mass and likely muscle strength appears to be a primary determinant of high-intensity exercise capacity. In a nutshell, getting stronger, although there may be no increase in muscle mass, will improve high-intensity exercise capacity of 4–7 minutes in duration. Clearly, overtraining in children should be avoided. In my opinion, more research effort (approved by institutional human subjects review committees) needs to be put forth on intense training in children, so coaches know where to draw the line as far as pushing kids too far. In addition, there should be more emphasis on coaching certifications so that coaches know where to draw the line as far as pushing kids too far. Logically, overtraining in children may stunt their growth and impair their ability to perform cognitive tasks in school.

Another way to train for Anaerobic Capacity is via 2–3 minute intervals at ~100% of VO_2 max. Medbo et al. (1988), Medbo and Tabata(1993) reported the best way to determine anaerobic capacity was by having subjects cycle for 2–3 minutes to exhaustion. This corresponds to about 100% of VO_2peak or max. It follows that this would be an excellent way to train for anaerobic capacity.

TRAINING FOR OPTIMAL AEROBIC CAPACITY AND CRITICAL POWER DURING THE SEASON

For wrestlers there are generally two reasons to train aerobically. One is to burn calories and keep their weight down. Thus, running, stationary cycling, and other aerobic type activities allow you to exercise for long periods of time and burn many calories. The other major reason is to exercise at intensities that approximate a wrestling match (95%–100% of VO_2max; Lambert and Jones 2010) and develop the cardiovascular system to a high degree for the physiological demands of a match. Clearly, at 100% of VO_2max you are stressing the cardiovascular system to a great degree. So you need to train the cardiovascular system so it adapts. The former reason (calorie burning) requires exercise for 20–60 minutes at a relatively moderate level of VO_2 (70% of VO_2max). The latter reason (getting the cardiovascular system in wrestling match shape) requires exercise for 6–7 minutes at or near VO_2max after a thorough warm up. This follows the SAID principle of specific adaptations to imposed demands or you get the adaptations you train for. Thus, specific training. Additionally, aerobic intervals of 5–10 minutes at the highest intensity you can maintain for 5–10 minutes will develop VO_2max, i.e., the maximal amount of oxygen that the respiratory, cardiovascular system can deliver to the muscles and the maximal amount of oxygen that can be used at the cellular level. The length of the rest period between intervals should be probably 2–3 minutes to allow recovery between bouts as exercise at VO_2max cannot be sustained indefinitely. The frequency of the aerobic training for wrestling should be 3–5 days/week. This is variable and dependent on the total training load on the student-athlete (see "Physiological Assessment and Determination of Overtraining" chapter).

TRAINING FOR AEROBIC CAPACITY IN THE OFF-SEASON

For improvements and maintenance of aerobic capacity in the off-season a good plan is to do your aerobic training 3 days a week for 30–60 minutes at a moderate intensity (60%–75% of VO_2max). This volume and intensity should allow enough recovery for optimal gains from your strength training.

It should be noted that there are conversions from heart rate max to VO_2max so the use of heart rate monitors is warranted.

COOL DOWN

A cool down should consist of 5–10 minutes of low to moderate intensity cardiovascular and muscular endurance activities (ACSM 2014).

TRAINING FOR MUSCULAR ENDURANCE

Generally speaking, the adaptations in muscle that accompany aerobic exercise training lead to an increase in muscular endurance. These adaptations include changes in the muscle fiber composition or fiber type from fast to slow, a change in the capillary density, a change in the myoglobin content, a change in the mitochondrial number and function, and a change in the amount of oxidative enzymes (Wilmore and Costill 1994). Additional adaptations are increases in lactic acid removal and oxidation (Brooks, Fahey, and Baldwin 2005) and an increase in muscle buffering capacity. Another positive adaptation with aerobic exercise training is an increase in the rate of ATP restoration after exercise (Kent-Braun, McCully, and Chance 1990).

TRAINING IN THE HEAT

Heat acclimatization (hot wrestling rooms) although it may expand plasma volume over time, as well as increase mental toughness, and improve performance in a normal temperature environment (Wilmore and Costill 1994), may be having the wrestlers concentrate on losing water weight rather than wrestling. However, if wrestlers must compete in a hot environment then at least part of their training should be conducted in a hot environment from a safety standpoint and for optimizing performance in a hot environment. Wrestling well and concentrating on the things that allow one to wrestle well such as technique, strength, anaerobic capacity, and aerobic capacity are more important than dehydration in the heat and clearly less dangerous. Further research is warranted to determine if training in a hot environment improves performance in a cool environment.

CONCURRENT TRAINING FOR STRENGTH AND ENDURANCE: THE RESEARCH AND BEYOND

The early studies on concurrent training, that is maximally training for both strength and endurance, suggest that endurance exercise impairs strength gains (Hickson 1980). This makes sense as training for fast myosin is optimal when training intensity is high and training frequency is low while training for slow myosin is optimal when training intensity is low and training frequency is high. Additionally, experienced Powerlifters only train as heavy as they can once per week while experienced Endurance Athletes train at a submaximal pace of 5–6 days per week. The question arises then as what should you do if you need both strength and endurance such as an amateur wrestler. It appears that you cannot optimize strength while training for endurance at a high frequency. One approach would be to reduce the number of times you train per week specifically for endurance. Additional evidence suggests that training for strength will augment your short-duration muscular endurance (i.e., endurance for 3–5 minutes at Peak VO_2; Lambert et al. (2013). Additionally, it appears that muscle mass per se has a bigger influence on VO_2 peak than previously thought (Lambert et al. 2020). Therefore, balancing your training time percentage-wise with more time than is typical going toward strength training and less time than is typical going toward endurance training may be a prudent move.

KEY POINTS

1. Strength training should be progressive in nature; if you get stronger, add weight; when you reach a plateau, switch routines, and always keep correct form on the exercises.
2. To train for maximal power (work/time), still train at slow speeds but intend to move the weight fast, since the research is equivocal on this point and slow speeds are less likely to get you injured.
3. To train for anaerobic capacity, train with 30-second to 1-minute intervals.
4. To train for maximal aerobic capacity train with intervals lasting 5–10 minutes each.
5. Training for muscular endurance is much like training for optimal aerobic capacity with 5–10 minute intervals but also training with long slow-distance aerobic work.
6. If wrestlers are going to compete in the heat than by all means train in the heat otherwise, avoid hot wrestling rooms. There is little if any research to support training hot and competing cool.
7. Concurrent training (Strength and Endurance training) optimally (i.e., good progress in both strength and endurance) may mean increasing the time spent resistance training and reducing the number of sessions of purely endurance or aerobic exercise.

15 Periodization

Periodization should consist of a 2–3 month, pre-season phase where athletes are lifting heavy weights and running long slow distance, followed by a competitive phase where there are three 4 week microcycles comprising 3 weeks of increased volume and 1 week of decreased volume. Microcycles should be progressively increased in volume over the course of 3 weeks and 3 months. This then should be followed by tapering phase of 3–4 weeks before major competitions at the end of the season. If wrestlers are competing in wrestling events in the "Off-Season" they should keep the scheme listed above in addition to wrestling in usually Freestyle and Greco-Roman competitions.

For amateur wrestling periodization for high-school student athletes it is broken down into a Pre-Season Phase lasting 2–3 months, a Competitive Season Phase lasting 3 months, and a peaking phase lasting 3–4 weeks in which a taper can be performed.

PRE-SEASON PHASE

During the Pre-Season Phase wrestlers should be losing fat with diet and long slow-distance aerobic exercise and should be strength training with low repetitions (3–6 per set) and attempting to get their body fat down to obtain an optimal strength-bodyweight ratio (Lambert and Jones 2010).

COMPETITIVE SEASON PHASE

During this phase the wrestler should be maintaining bodyweight and eating to train (Lambert and Jones 2010) and training to improve the amount of work they can accomplish during a training session and a match. During this phase weightlifting should be once per week per muscle group. Drilling should be conducted 3–4 times per week and 15–20 minutes per session. Aerobic exercise should be conducted 3–4 times per week. I would suggest one long slow-distance run to maintain bodyweight between 30–60 minutes duration. Additionally, for specificity according to the Specific Adaptations to Imposed Demands (SAID) principle, one 6 minute run for distance should be conducted per week, and one 15 minute run for distance should be conducted as well during the week. With regard to live wrestling, the goal should be to increase the amount of work a wrestler can do throughout the season. For this I would suggest a summated microcycle (Stone and Stone 2008). This would be a 3/1 summated microcycle with 3 weeks of increased volume of live wrestling (time) and 1 week of reduced volume (time) performed three or four times over the course of the competitive season. The intensity stays the same at maximal effort. Live wrestling should be the basis of in-season strength and conditioning and should correspond to about 60%–75% of total practice time with drilling, lifting, and aerobic conditioning conducted for the remaining 25%–40% of the time. According to Stone and Stone (2008) an appropriate reduction in volume (time) during the recovery weeks would be 10%, 20%, 25%, and 30% reduction in training volume during the 4th week of the 3/1 microcycle. The idea behind this is that the amount of work will be increased at a given intensity (maximal "Go's") by increasing the time. The idea behind the recovery week is to allow for recovery and supercompensation from the prior microcycle and to prevent overtraining. Each 3 week part of the microcycle will have greater volume than the previous one.

With the information in the previous block being proposed; utilization of some measure of overtraining would be useful. These are detailed in the following chapter.

TAPERING FOR OPTIMAL PERFORMANCE

For improvements in performance near the end of the season it is important that the coach has the athletes taper. This is a lessening in the volume of the work over time but a maintenance of intensity of work, traditionally. In running, Shepley et al. (1992) found that a low-volume high-intensity taper led to a 22% improvement in 1,500 m performance. The duration of the taper was 7 days. Houmard et al. (1994) also found that a low-volume high-intensity taper was beneficial to 5 k run time (3% improvement) and improved running economy or a reduced oxygen cost of standardized submaximal exercise by 7%.

Gibala, MacDougall, and Sale (1994) found that a high-intensity low-volume taper improved strength training performance over 8 days compared to a rest only taper. Trappe, Costill, and Thomas (2000) examined the effects of a 21 day taper after 5 months of high-volume, high-intensity training. Swim power increased 15% on a swim power bench and swim performance was improved by 4%. This was measured by an increase in the size of the Type IIa and Type I fibers and improvement in the speed of contraction of the Type IIB fibers (67%).

Clearly, there is a benefit of a high-intensity low-volume 3 week taper on high-intensity exercise performance. For an excellent book on the topic of tapering see Mujika (2009).

If wrestlers are competing in competitions in the "Off-Season" they should keep this schema for the six to seven months as described above. Clearly, it is not a prudent practice to take the three to four months that are not scheduled in this schema off from resistance training or aerobic exercise training as deconditioning of strength and aerobic attributes can occur. Deconditioning from aerobic exercise can happen in as little as a week of inactivity (Shoemaker et al. 1998) (Tables 15.1 and 15.2).

TABLE 15.1
Six to Eight Month Training Plan

Phase	Duration	Focus
Pre-season	2–3 months	Strength accumulation (improving maximal instantaneous power output) and fat loss
Competitive season	3 months (broken down into 3 microcycles: 3 weeks of increase in volume, followed by 1 deload week)	Weight maintenance, muscle mass maintenance, fueling training appropriately, and improving (whole match power output)
Peaking	3–4 weeks	Tapering to optimize aerobic and anaerobic performance

TABLE 15.2
Purpose, Training, and Nutrition for the Six-Eight Month Plan

Phases of Training	Pre-Competitive (2–3 months)	Competitive (3–4 months)	Peaking/Tapering (1 month)
Purpose	Gain strength and lose fat	Maintain strength and improve entire match power output	Taper for peak performance at local, regional, state, and national tournaments
Training	Resistance training 3–6 Reps, 4×/week Long Slow Distance 3–5×/week	Live wrestling Drilling Resistance training Intense aerobic and anaerobic exercise	Reduced volume each week and maintain intensity
Nutrition	High protein (>1.6 g/kg/day, Moderate carbohydrate, low fat. Stay in negative energy balance by about 20% to lose 1–2 lbs/week	60 CHO, 20 PRO, 20 FAT (8–10 g/kg/day CHO, 1.5 g/kg/day PRO, 0.7 g/kg/day fat; stay in energy balance	60 CHO, 20 PRO, 20 FAT (8–10 g/kg/day CHO, 1.5 g/kg/day PRO, 0.7 g/kg/day fat; stay in energy balance or slightly +energy balance

KEY POINTS

1. Training during the Pre-season Phase should be for 2–3 months and heavy weightlifting should be undertaken along with long slow-distance aerobic training.
2. A good way for training during the Competitive Phase which last three months consists of three 4 week microcycles of 3 weeks of heavy training, each of increasing volume, and each followed by a dload week. (deload).
3. The tapering phase consists of 3–4 weeks of reducing volume while increasing or maintaining intensity over the course of 3–4 weeks.
4. Varying training load and especially tapering are *ESSENTIAL* for the success of competitive wrestlers. These concepts need to become part of every Wrestling Coach's vocabulary.

16 Physiological Assessment and Determination of Overtraining

Training stress should be assessed to determine progress, lack thereof, and whether the athlete is overtrained or not. The Cooper 12-minute run can be used to assess aerobic capacity, the Wingate Anaerobic Test, and time to fatigue at 100% of VO_2max/peak can be used to assess anaerobic capacity, while maximal strength testing on the three Powerlifts can be used to determine maximal strength. These tests should be used about every three to four weeks to assess training status. Overtraining is a stagnation of training progress and has many physical symptoms such as weight loss and a reduction in appetite, lethargy, and upper respiratory tract infections (URTI). A number of strategies can be employed to stave off overtraining collectively known as good training hygiene. Overtraining can be assessed by the Daily Analysis of Life Demands in Athletes (DALDA) questionnaire which is the (DALDA), Profile of Mood States (POMS), practice Ratings of Perceived Exertion (RPE), various sleep questionnaires, blood lactate, and blood glucose measurements. Also, the potential for Relative Energy Deficiency in Sport should be assessed and clearly the Coaches should track metrics on these indexes throughout the season.

Physiological and psychological assessment over the course of the season would appear to be extremely important in determining if you are improving and by how much, if you are staying the same, or if your conditioning is regressing. Assessments should be made every 3 weeks during the season on the same day and at the same time of day. Examples of ways to assess performance during the season as well as ways to monitor training status and prevent overtraining are listed below.

COOPER 12-MINUTE TEST FOR ASSESSING MAXIMAL FITNESS LEVEL (VO₂max)

Field tests such as the Cooper 12-minute test (1968) are a great alternative to getting your VO_2max tested in the laboratory. This is important as VO_2max is a very important measure of wrestling fitness as wrestling is conducted at 95%–100% of VO_2max (Lambert and Jones 2010). For the Cooper 12-minute test you need a timer, a stop watch, and a 400 m track. The athlete runs for 12-minutes and the distance in meters is determined to the nearest 10 m (estimated). A warm up precedes the test, of course. For a detailed way to calculate VO_2max from the distance covered in meters, please see *www.brianmac.co.uk*. As discussed above VO_2max is the single best measure of aerobic fitness level. This test can be used to assess VO_2max throughout the season and determine progress throughout the season. This test probably should be done every three weeks to once a month.

WINGATE ANAEROBIC TEST FOR ARMS AND LEGS

Another test you can use to examine progress over the course of the season (probably about every three or four weeks) is the Wingate Anaerobic Test for Arms and Legs. With this test you can obtain Peak Power, Average Power, Total Work, and a fatigue index. It involves "all out" cycling on a cycle ergometer for 30 seconds with a load on the bike equivalent to 0.075 kg/kg body weight on a Monark Cycle Ergometer (Dotan and Bar-Or 1983). Links to the software are available for a Monark Cycle Ergometer from www.monarkexercise.se. You should perform this test for both arms and legs. It is a great test of anaerobic capabilities.

TIME TO FATIGUE AT ~100% OF VO$_2$ peak

Medbo et al. (1988), Medbo and Tabata (1993) determined that having subjects' cycle for about 2–3 minute to exhaustion and determine the distance covered under a standardized situation was an excellent way to determine anaerobic capacity. It follows that performing a time to fatigue test about once a month at about 100% of VO$_2$ max (same power output each time you test) would be an excellent way to determine whether anaerobic capacity is getting better, staying the same, or getting worse over the course of training.

STRENGTH TESTING THROUGHOUT THE SEASON

Monitoring strength is very important over the course of the season to see where the athlete is; either staying the same, gaining, or losing strength. These changes in muscular strength could be due to training, recovery, and/or nutritional status. You should monitor your progress probably every three weeks by performing maximal Bench Press, Squat, and Deadlift over the course of the season, and these can be done on lifting days. Clearly, if you are losing strength the coach and athlete need to do something about it with regard to reducing the intensity or volume of training sessions, increasing protein and/or carbohydrate consumption, and/or increasing recovery time between workouts. As little as a 5 lbs drop in strength is an important drop and should be dealt with. Make sure the lifts are done when the athlete is fresh and not fatigued from practice.

OVERTRAINING

Overtraining is a reduction in physiological performance brought on by a prolonged increase in training load. It is accompanied by a number of physiological signs and symptoms. Overtraining can occur from a lack of sufficient carbohydrate intake which results in glycogen depletion when training intensity and volume are high. Costill et al. (1988) reported that an intensified period of collegiate swim training resulted in a reduction of performance. A further analysis of the data revealed that the swimmers who could not maintain the desired intensity for the given volume of training were not eating sufficient carbohydrate and had low muscle glycogen concentrations. These data are supported in runners by Kirwan et al. (1988), who found that even 10 g of carbohydrate per kilogram body weight was insufficient to maintain running performance during a period of intensified training. For a remedy to this form of overtraining please see Lambert and Jones (2010). Clearly, eating insufficient carbohydrate can lead to overtraining but overtraining can occur in the face of sufficient carbohydrate intake (Snyder et al. 1995). According to Wilmore and Costill (1994) the symptoms of overtraining are as follows (Table 16.1).

These symptoms of overtraining, however, are highly individualized according to Wilmore and Costill (1994).

URTI AND EXERCISE

The risk of URTIs and exercise is quite interesting. No exercise training and you have an average risk of a URTI, moderate exercise training and you have a lower than average risk of an URTI. If you train excessively you have an above average risk of an URTI (Nieman 1997). Thus, excessive training will likely give you an URTI. In an excellent article in the *Journal of Athletic Training*, Nieman (1997) describes that the risk of an URTI is doubled for a runner who runs ~60 miles per week (~8.6 miles/day) compared with a runner who runs ~20 miles/week (~2.9 miles/day). This investigator also described eight precautions that will reduce the risk of an URTI (Table 16.2).

The use of carbohydrate beverages to assist with optimal immune system function is supported by the work of McFarlin et al. (2004) from another excellent group of researchers.

MONITORING OVERTRAINING

Ways to monitor overtraining include use of the POMS, the DALDA questionnaire, and RPE (see below) and blood glucose and blood lactic acid testing.

THE DAILY ANALYSIS OF LIFE DEMANDS IN ATHLETES (DALDA)

The DALDA can be used to monitor overtraining. After a period of baseline assessment, use the DALDA questionnaire to determine the frequency of worse than

---

TABLE 16.1

Symptoms of Overtraining

Weight loss and a reduction in appetite

Muscle soreness

Colds and allergic reactions

Nausea occasionally

Disturbances in sleep

Elevated resting heart rate and blood pressure

TABLE 16.2
Factors that Reduce the Risk of URTIs

1. Eating a well-balanced diet and adding a Vitamin C supplement may be helpful
2. Reduce other life stressors such as mental stress
3. Do not overtrain
4. Do not lose more than 1% of bodyweight per week
5. Do not put your hands in your eyes or nose, stay away from sick people, and stay away from large crowds before competitions
6. Flu shots are recommended for heavy training athletes
7. Get adequate sleep
8. Use carbohydrate beverages before, during, and after heavy training such as marathon training. You may not think this is applicable but the world record for the marathon is just less than two hours. How long do your practices last?

normal fatigue scores. Five or more worse than normal fatigue scores for four consecutive days (this means daily measurements) mean you should recover or decrease the intensity and/or volume of your workouts or other stressors. Any easy way to do this is graph number of fatigue scores (worse than normal) on Y axis and days on the X axis. This can be done with paper and pencil or with a computer program such as Excel (Rushall 1990; Halson and Jones 2002) (Table 16.3).

POMS (AVAILABLE FROM www.brianmac.co.uk)

The POMS consists of 65 adjectives which are rated by the participants on a five point scale. These 65 adjectives form six factors: tension-anxiety, depression-dejection, anger-hostility, fatigue-inertia, vigor-activity, and confusion-bewilderment. The optimal mood state is obviously obtained when tension-anxiety, depression-dejection, anger-hostility, fatigue-inertia, and confusion-bewilderment are low and vigor-activity are high. Clearly when one is overtrained or stale this is the case. This could be tracked weekly over a baseline period and during the season to determine overtraining or staleness. A computer program to take the POMS and get your scores is available at www.brianmac.co.uk.

RATING OF PERCEIVED EXERTION (BORG; AVAILABLE FROM my.clevelandclinic.org/rpe-scale-heart-health)

This is another tool which can be used to determine staleness or the overtrained state. It is simply a subjective measure of how the athlete perceived the training session or part of a training session. It can be tracked over the season. For example, if the same practices are conducted with an increase in the perceived exertion this likely is a measure on an overtrained state. Again, this is due to glycogen depletion or an overtrained state despite normal muscle glycogen concentrations (Costill et al. 1988; Snyder et al. 1995).

TABLE 16.3
DALDA Questionnaire

Part A

1. A B C Diet
2. A B C Home life
3. A B C School/college/work
4. A B C Friends
5. A B C Sport training
6. A B C Climate
7. A B C Sleep
8. A B C Recreation
9. A B C Health

Part B

1. A B C Muscle pains	14. A B C Enough sleep
2. A B C Techniques	15. A B C Between-session recovery
3. A B C Tiredness	16. A B C General weakness
4. A B C Need for a rest	17. A B C Interest
5. A B C Supplementary work	18. A B C Arguments
6. A B C Boredom	19. A B C Skin rashes
7. A B C Recovery time	20. A B C Congestion
8. A B C Irritability	21. A B C Training effort
9. A B C Weight	22. A B C Temper
10. A B C Throat	23. A B C Swellings
11. A B C Internal	24. A B C Likability
12. A B C Unexplained aches	25. A B C Runny nose
13. A B C Technique strength	

Source: Available at fullsus.co.za/dalda-questionnaire/.
A = worse than normal.
B = normal.
C = better than normal.
Rushall (1990).

TESTING FOR BLOOD GLUCOSE AND BLOOD LACTIC ACID CONCENTRATION

Testing for blood glucose and blood lactic acid although not commonly done in collegiate or high-school wrestling is often done in collegiate swimming. Blood glucose can be used to determine if a wrestler is hypoglycemic and the extent of liver glycogen depletion. During intense exercise liver glycogen is broken down to blood glucose and glucose in the blood becomes elevated. As time goes on the muscle uptake of the glucose that is dumped into the blood reduces the blood glucose concentration. If carbohydrate is not taken in sufficient quantities, the wrestler will become hypoglycemic. This is a critically low level of blood glucose and a good measure of total body carbohydrate stores being way too low. Blood lactic acid levels during exercise of the same intensity is taken during exercise of the same high intensity on two or more occasions are an indicator of muscle glycogen concentrations. Low glycogen results in low blood lactate (lactic acid) production and accumulation in the blood (during the initial portion of intense exercise). Clearly, these two measures would be important for determining the nutritional status of the wrestlers and the extent to which a given practice alters these variables.

THE IMPORTANCE OF SLEEP TO OPTIMAL TRAINING AND RECOVERY

It is clear that adequate amounts and quality of sleep are important to physiological performance and recovery. A recent study in collegiate basketball players illustrates this fact. Mah et al. (2011) reported that 41.5 days of sleep extension (they slept longer each night) by approximately 110 minutes per night from 7.8–10.4 hours per night had a clear positive effect on reaction time (Psychomotor Vigilance Task), sprinting speed, free throw percentage, three point field goal percentage, as well as the players subjective self-rating for practices and games. Additionally, scores on the Epworth Sleep Scale and POMS improved significantly as a result of sleep extension. Clearly, increasing the time an athlete sleeps by a couple of hours per night can have a profound impact on physiological and psychological measures pertinent to the sport in question (Mah et al. 2011). It follows that sleep extension would likely be beneficial for amateur wrestlers of all ages and performance capabilities.

USE OF SLEEP SCALES

Two such scales are the Pittsburgh Sleep Quality Inventory based on the previous section, which may be beneficial to track as a metric the sleep quality and quantity (PSQI; Available on the internet via Google) and the Epworth Sleepiness Scale (ESS; Available on the internet via Google). As indicated in the titles the PSQI measures sleep quality and the ESS measures daytime sleepiness. Clearly, in hard training wrestlers who are also possibly restricting energy (calorie) intake, sleep quality, and duration could be disrupted. Additionally, from personal experience and logic it would follow that daytime sleepiness could be a problem for wrestlers who are both training hard and studying. As a result, monitoring your athletes sleep would appear to be beneficial from both an academic and athletic standpoint.

TRACKING METRICS FOR WRESTLING

Clearly it would be important for coaches to track metrics during the wrestling season. There are no commercially available programs to track metrics specifically for wrestling training, to my knowledge. My suggestion would be to use Microsoft Excel or track these metrics with a lab notebook and a pencil. On the X axis would be days of training and on the Y axis would be the metric you were interested in. Metrics which could be tracked on a daily or weekly basis could be DALDA scores, POMS scores, sprint times, weightlifting data, weight, calorie intake, carbohydrate intake, and protein intake. Clearly, this would be a time and effort intensive undertaking by any coaching staff but it may be well worth the time and effort from the standpoint of wrestling and academic performance. The art of coaching would be to determine which combination of metrics would result in a dip in wrestling and academic performance over the course of the season. This would also take a bit of effort on the part of the student-athlete to track their metrics to give to the coach.

KEY POINT

1. Overtraining is a widespread problem in sports. Monitoring training stress is very important and can be done using objective physiological measures and subjective questionnaire information. Regardless, the more carefully collected the information, a greater quantity of it will help to monitor training stress and optimize performance to a great extent (Tables 16.4 and 16.5).

TABLE 16.4
Objective Methods for Monitoring Training Progress

Test (Every 3–4 weeks)	Purpose	Advantages/Disadvantages
Cooper 12-minute run test	To assess VO_2max or in other words Max Aerobic Fitness	Easy to administer/may add to training load
Wingate 30-second anaerobic test	To assess anaerobic parameters	Need a special stationary bike (Monark) but easy to administer/adds little to training load
Time to fatigue at 100% VO_2peak	To assess aerobic and anaerobic capacities	Need to assess VO_2peak/max. Takes 3–6 minutes, may add to training load
Blood glucose and blood lactate	Used to assess fitness level and nutritional status	Specialized equipment required and finger stick blood sampling/provides useful objective information
Strength testing	Assess strength throughout the season to monitor training, nutrition, and rest	Simple to perform, does not add to training load. Great information about the overall condition of your athletes

TABLE 16.5

Subjective Methods for Monitoring Training Progress

Test (Daily)	Purpose	Advantages/Disadvantages
DALDA questionnaire	Assess overall health and well-being of the athlete including psychology	Gives both good physiologic and psychologic feedback. Designed for exercise training/frequency of admin
POMS	Assesses the psychological mood of the athlete which appears to be directly influenced by physiology	A good measure and relatively easy to use/frequency of admin
RPE	Assesses the perception of effort during a practice	Ease of use. Student-athlete self-report/ frequency of admin
Sleep scales	Assess the quality and quantity of sleep	Important information for recovery/a bit cumbersome and frequency of admin

Part 2

Nutrition for Amateur Wrestling
Fueling the Machine

17 Amateur Wrestling Nutrition and Metabolism Primer

Metabolism can be broken down into Anabolism or building up reactions and Catabolism or breaking down reactions. Carbohydrates are the primary fuel for high-intensity exercise such as wrestling which can is be typically done at 100% of VO$_2$max. Proteins and amino acids provide the building blocks for post post-exercise muscle protein synthesis while fats are important for the absorption of the fat soluble vitamins. Many vitamins provide co-factors for the metabolic reactions while minerals provide the electrolytes for muscle contraction and nerve conduction.

AMATEUR WRESTLING NUTRITION AND METABOLISM PRIMER

DEFINITIONS

This first chapter will deal with the basics of nutrition and metabolism as they relate to amateur wrestling. The meaning of nutrition is quite easy … it is just what we eat. Nutrition is the intake of carbohydrates, proteins, lipids, vitamins, minerals, and water. The definition of metabolism, however, is more complicated. Metabolism is the sum total of all of the chemical reactions in the body and is made up of anabolism and catabolism (Stryer 1988).

ANABOLISM AND CATABOLISM (STRYER 1988)

Anabolism is the building up of a large structural component of the body from smaller "building blocks". Catabolism is the breaking down of large structural components stored in the muscle and other organs into smaller subunits such as the breakdown of glycogen (stored carbohydrate) to glucose (usable carbohydrate). Obvious examples of anabolic processes in the body deal with the building up of carbohydrate (glycogen from glucose), protein (protein from amino acids), and fat (adipose tissue from fatty acids and glycerol) in the body from their building blocks. Carbohydrate stores, also known as glycogen, found in muscle and liver, are built up from glucose subunits, and this is an **anabolic process**. Glucose is the sugar that all ingested carbohydrate is broken down to by the gastrointestinal tract, and this glucose enters into the blood from the gastrointestinal tract. Individual glucose molecules then go to the liver and muscle and are linked together in the muscle and liver to form larger branched glycogen molecules, the storage form of carbohydrate in the body called glycogen. When we need glucose in the blood because blood glucose is low, for example, in the fasted state, *liver* glycogen is broken down to glucose which is released into the blood. When we need energy for muscle contraction at a high rate and the duration of exercise is greater than a few seconds *muscle* glycogen is broken down for energy (adenosine triphosphate (ATP)) and to provide phosphorylated glucose to make more energy. Both of these situations, in liver and in muscle, are *catabolic processes*. With regard to protein, structural proteins within the body which formulate muscle tissue used in muscle contractions are built up from amino acids that come from the breakdown of proteins we eat in food. These amino acids from food are then delivered in the blood to the muscle where structural proteins are built up from the ingested amino acids. This is an *anabolic process*. During prolonged aerobic exercise (up to 20% of the needs of the exercise; Lemon et al. 1992), and during fasting, proteins from muscle tissue and liver are broken down to amino acids, and the amino acids are utilized for energy (the amino nitrogen from the amino acids is converted to urea which is then released into the urine, and we can use the carbon that is left over for energy just like the carbon from carbohydrates). This is a *catabolic process*. Fat metabolism is to some extent more complicated but in essence involves building up fat stores under the skin, around our organs, and in muscle from fatty acids and glycerol that are the components of fat that we ingest, which is an *anabolic process*. During lower intensity and more prolonged exercise than wrestling as well as during fasting, fats are broken down to their components and can be utilized for energy, which is a *catabolic process*.

NUTRITIONAL COMPONENTS AND WRESTLING SUCCESS

Macronutrients: Carbohydrates, Protein, and Fat.

CARBOHYDRATE

Carbohydrates are made of carbon, hydrogen, and water and in multiples of CH_2O. Carbohydrates primarily serve the role of providing energy and especially during exercise. They also can serve structural role, for example cellulose which is in the structure of the plant cell wall. The most simple carbohydrates are called monosaccharides and are made of one sugar molecule. These include glucose, fructose, and galactose. Glucose is found in blood, and all carbohydrates are ultimately broken down into glucose by the liver if they are to be used for the production of ATP in liver or skeletal muscle. Fructose is found in fruit, and its derivative high-fructose corn syrup is found in pop and sodas. Fructose goes to the liver and is converted to glucose, and there when ingested by itself, fructose raises blood glucose levels slower than glucose or maltodextrins which are multiple glucoses bonded end to end. Galactose is found in milk and with glucose forms lactose or milk sugar. Galactose is broken down into glucose by the liver, also. Other disaccharides besides lactose are sucrose or table sugar, maltose, and isomaltose. Maltose is two glucoses bonded together and isomaltose is two glucoses bonded together in branch configuration. The third class of carbohydrates are the polysaccharides which are many sugars bonded end to end. One such polysaccharide is maltodextrin which is glucoses bonded end to end. Another important polysaccharide from the standpoint of exercise is glycogen which is glucoses strung together in a branching configuration. Glycogen is stored in liver and skeletal muscle and provides glucose for buffering blood glucose concentrations, i.e., raising them when they are low. The glycogen found in skeletal muscle gets broken down to glucose-1-phosphate, then glucose-6-phosphate, and can be used to make limited amounts of ATP (3 ATP) without oxygen (anaerobic glycolysis to lactate) or can used to make an abundant amount of ATP via *aerobic* glycolysis to acetyl-CoA which when it enters the Krebs Cycle allows for an abundant amount of ATP to be made (~39 ATP). Clearly, when oxygen is available more ATP can be made; however, it is made at a slower rate than that can be made without oxygen. Without carbohydrates you cannot perform intense exercise. Let me clarify, you can perform intense exercise but at much lower power outputs trying to use pure fat than by using carbohydrate rather than fat (McCartney et al. 1986). During a wrestling match, carbohydrates are by far the most important source of energy. Very little fat and protein are utilized during a match, and if they are being used predominantly your power output will go down. The intensity of exercise that a wrestling match is competed at is, on average, ~100% of VO_2max (Gleeson, Greenhaff, and Maughan 1988). At that intensity of exercise, stored carbohydrate (muscle glycogen) provides almost all of the energy (Gollnick et al. 1973). Other important sources of fuel are stored ATP () and phosphocreatine (PC) in the muscle. However, these stored sources run out within the first 30 seconds or less of the match (Wilmore and Costill 1994). Therefore, carbohydrates are the next available fuel source in sequence for providing energy during exercise. At the severity of effort that wrestlers compete at 95%–100% of VO_2max it has been estimated that ~99% of the energy needs are derived from muscle glycogen and ~1% is derived from blood glucose (Katz et al. 1986), and it must be noted that these data were obtained in untrained subjects. Slightly greater amounts of blood glucose could be used oxidatively or non-oxidatively in trained individuals exercising high intensities relative to the amount of glycogen used anaerobically. How much we don't know. Likely more than 1% of the total carbohydrate is utilized. Very little if any fat is utilized *during a match*. There is at least 50 years of solid research supporting a major role for a high-carbohydrate diet and/or carbohydrate feedings during exercise in improving exercise performance when muscle glycogen is the major source of energy (Below et al. 1995; Bergstrom et al. 1967; Bergstrom and Hultman 1967; Coggan and Coyle 1987; Costill et al. 1973; Foster, Costill, and Fink 1979, Karlsson and Saltin 1971; Little et al. 2009; Mitchell et al. 1988, 1989; Neufer et al. 1987; Sherman et al. 1981).

PROTEIN AND AMINO ACIDS

Protein is made up of amino acids. Proteins have a myriad of functions within the human body. The sole function of our DNA is to code for proteins, and proteins make everything else. Clearly, having adequate protein in the diet is of paramount importance for these reasons. One must remember that protein requirements change with activity level and age. Proteins are made up of Amino Acids. Amino acids are made up of carbon, hydrogen, oxygen, and nitrogen. The amino acids are bonded together in many different structural configurations to make proteins (more than 100 amino acids). There are 20 different amino acids, of which 10 are considered essential amino acids. Essential amino acids must be provided in the diet while the other 10 are non-essential amino acids that can be synthesized from each other. Amino acids have an amino group, a carboxyl group, a hydrogen, and R-group. The R-group makes each of the 20 different amino acids different, i.e., each one has a different structural makeup. You will note that the presence of nitrogen makes amino acids different than carbohydrates and fats which do have carbon, hydrogen, and oxygen but not nitrogen. In fact, in times of energy lack, i.e., negative energy balance meaning dieting with a low protein diet, the amino acids from proteins within the body are utilized for energy. That is the nitrogen groups are lopped off and form urea by way of the liver and are excreted in the urine (giving a very pungent smelling urine), and carbon skeleton can be used like a carbohydrate. The utilization of protein and amino acids as an energy source *during* a match is unlikely as Lemon and co-workers reported that protein utilization during optimal conditions for protein oxidation only was ~20% during prolonged submaximal exercise. This is likely because of the complicated processes involved in the degradation of protein, the deamination of amino acids, and the transport and oxidation of the carbon skeleton by skeletal muscle. Clearly, being in negative protein balance will lead to muscle loss while that also is the case for negative energy balance but to a lesser extent if you are taking in a lot of protein. Interestingly, the work of Rennie's group (Bowtell et al. 2000) shows that the ingestion of carbohydrate (glucose specifically) will reduce amino acid oxidation during exercise. This would be considered a positive thing for the athlete. It is impossible to lose weight in a positive energy balance. It is also likely that lean body mass will be lost when one attempts to lose fat. Ideally, one would lose weight before the season on a higher protein reduced energy diet when the energy (carbohydrate) demands of training are not so great. During the season, adequate energy (carbohydrate energy) for glycogen resynthesis, protein (above the RDA) for muscle protein resynthesis, fat (probably at least 50 g/day), fluid, and vitamins and minerals should be consumed, but the importance of protein and amino acids are that they are primarily the building blocks for muscle repair and rebuilding after an intense bout of exercise such as a resistance training session or a wrestling workout. Additionally, proteins and amino acids are important for the immune system and maintenance of fluid volume within the plasma compartment of the cardiovascular system.

FAT

Lipids or fat are very important in the human body. Most fats, i.e., triglycerides, are used for energy storage. The second most abundant type of fat is a phospholipid which is found in all of our cell membranes and makes the phospholipid bilayer. Third are steroids which have a cholesterol ring within them and are sex hormones such as testosterone, estrogen, and progesterone. The fourth type of lipid is the Eicosanoids made up of Prostaglandins, Leukotrienes, and Thromboxanes.

We will focus our attention on triglycerides. The most abundant source of triglycerides is found in fat cells subcutaneously and around the organs (visceral fat depots). Additionally, triglycerides are stored within muscle cells as intramuscular triglycerides. Within the cell membrane of fat cells or adipocytes, hormone sensitive lipase acts to bind the hormone epinephrine and allow for the liberation of fatty acids and glycerol from the fat cell. The fatty acids can be used for oxidation by the skeletal muscle, and the glycerol potentially can go to the liver and be converted to glucose via gluconeogenesis. In the skeletal muscle triglycerides can be broken down into fatty acids and glycerol. The fatty acids can then be oxidized by the skeletal muscle, and glycerol can go out during the circulation and be delivered to the liver for conversion to glucose via gluconeogenesis. The liver forms many types of lipids including phospholipids, lipoproteins (HDL, LDL, VLDL), and triglycerides. Generally speaking, the Eicosanoids are used for inflammation. As stated previously, the utilization of fat during a single match is negligible, but the utilization of fat goes up as the number of matches in a row during practice goes up (McCartney et al. 1986). Also, you mobilize fat stores to obtain energy in the recovery period between matches in practice or competition. Additionally, the lower your muscle glycogen (carbohydrate) stores, the greater the utilization of fat. Unfortunately, if inadequate carbohydrate is available, and the reliance on fat goes up, **the intensity of exercise must be lowered, because fat provides energy too slowly compared to carbohydrates, which means lowered power output and reduced performance** (McCartney et al. 1986). Dietary fats are very important for the absorption of fat soluble vitamins: D, A, K, and E. Additionally, structural fats in the body makeup part of the cell membranes of all cells and the lining of cells of the nervous system are called myelin (Table 17.1).

VITAMINS AND MINERALS

Vitamins and minerals, the so-called "micronutrients", help to support immune function, muscle function, and are very important in almost all aspects of the buildup (anabolism) and breakdown (catabolism) of substances in the body (metabolism). The functions that vitamins and minerals perform are numerous. We will first start with the water soluble vitamins: Vitamin C is needed as an antioxidant and may help prevent upper respiratory tract infections during periods of extreme training. The B vitamins are, generally speaking, needed to break down carbohydrates for energy. With regard to fat soluble vitamins, Vitamins D, A, K, and E, they need to be taken with fat in the diet or they are not absorbed. Vitamin D-3 is important for muscle and bone health as well as the health of the immune system. Vitamin E also known

TABLE 17.1

Major Sources and Functions of the Macronutrients

Macronutrients	
Carbohydrates	Provide energy for rest and exercise. The predominant fuel for high-intensity exercise (80%–200% VO$_2$peak)
Protein	Provides the amino acids for muscle protein synthesis, forms some hormones, carrier proteins, and enzymes
Fats	Stored fats provide energy for low-moderate intensity exercise. Important for the absorption of Vitamins D, A, K, and E and some forms of hormones

as alpha-tocopherol is a strong antioxidant. Vitamin K is needed for blood clotting while vitamin A is necessary for the growth and development of most kinds of epithelial cells and also for the normal synthesis of retinal photochemicals. If taken in excess, fat soluble vitamins build up in the liver and can be toxic. With regard to the minerals, sodium, Na^+, and potassium, K^+, are required for normal muscle function including cardiac muscle. Magnesium, Mg^{2+}, is needed for the ability to use ATP during muscle contraction, while calcium, Ca^{2+}, is essential to maintain normal muscle contraction including cardiac muscle. Chloride, Cl^-, along with Na^+ is important for maintaining extracellular fluid volume. Needless to say, it is important to ingest adequate amounts of all of the essential vitamins and minerals. Attaining this adequate level of vitamins and minerals can be done most appropriately by eating a varied diet rich in fruits and vegetables of various different colors. Also, you can ensure that you are getting adequate vitamins and minerals by taking a complete multivitamin/mineral tablet daily. The importance of vitamins and minerals is great and not to be overlooked. You should try to obtain the Recommended Daily Allowance of all vitamins and minerals which may be difficult to do on a diet of 2,000 kcals or less.

TABLE OF FUNCTIONS OF VITAMINS AND MINERALS

INTERMEDIARY METABOLISM

The three major macronutrients Carbohydrates, Proteins, and Fats can produce an abundant amount of ATP when oxygen and time are available. Carbohydrates (namely Glycogen and Glucose) are broken down ultimately to Acetyl Co-A, which can then be fed into the Krebs Cycle and the Electron Transport Chain, and Oxidative Phosphorylation, to produce an abundant amount of ATP per glucose molecule (38–39 ATP). Fats (specifically triglycerides) can release fatty acids which can be converted to Acetyl Co-A and oxidized to produce large amounts of ATP per fatty acid (Palmitic Acid = 129 ATP; Wilmore and Costill 1994) after the acetyl Co-A goes through the Krebs Cycle, Electron Transport Chain, and Oxidative Phosphorylation. The glycerol from the triglyceride is glucogenic, meaning it can go to the liver and be converted to glucose via gluconeogenesis (the making of new glucose from noncarbohydrate sources). The Amino Acids from muscle protein or those ingested are quite unique in that _19_ amino acids can be used for gluconeogenesis in the liver while eight can go to Acetyl Co-A and be oxidized for ATP in the skeletal muscle likely for a similar amount of ATP as a glucose molecule. Amino acid oxidation, quantitatively, in skeletal muscle is at most ~20% during prolonged exercise (Lemon, Dolny, and Yarasheski 1997). Interestingly, Rennie's group (Bowtell et al. 2000) found that glucose ingestion during exercise reduced leucine oxidation by about 20% when protein intake was about 1.8 g/kg/day at 60% of VO_2max, suggesting that ingesting glucose during exercise will spare muscle protein.

KEY POINTS

1. Anabolism is building up reactions while catabolism is breaking down reactions.
2. Carbohydrates are stored as liver and muscle glycogen in anabolic reactions and released as blood glucose in a catabolic reaction. Blood glucose is the third storage source of carbohydrate. Carbohydrates are of primary importance for all types of exercise. A longstanding tenet of biochemistry is that fats burn in a carbohydrate flame; therefore, carbohydrates are essential for almost all durations and intensities of exercise.
3. Proteins are typically considered the result of anabolic reactions involving amino acids. Proteins can be utilized during periods of lack of carbohydrate for liberating amino acids, and utilization of these amino acids is through a process called gluconeogenesis. In individuals on a mixed diet (normal American diet), amino acid oxidation can account for about 20% of energy needs.
4. Fats can be utilized for energy at low exercise intensities in untrained individuals while trained individuals can utilize fats better than untrained, and this spares muscle and blood carbohydrate. Fats typically are not believed to be used at maximal intensities of exercise, unless possibly when the muscle glycogen stores are depleted. This, however, results in a drop in power output likely because of the oxygen requirement for fat combustion.
5. Vitamins and minerals are essential to normal function, and many are involved in anabolic and catabolic pathways involving energy metabolism.
6. It is important to note that carbohydrate intake during exercise spares muscle amino acids from being combusted. Clearly, an area of further research would compare the ability of carbohydrate and amino acid ingestion on muscle amino acid combustion.

18 Water Balance, Electrolyte Balance, and Hydration

Rapid weight loss can be dangerous as the death of three collegiate wrestlers in 1997 being evidence of this, although the ingestion of ephedrine based drinks may have played a role. Legislation brought forth by Senator John McCain resulted in the criminalization of ephedrine while the NCAA and High School Athletic Associations have instituted a number of safe practices for Weight Management. Such practices include hydration testing, body fat testing, and minimizing the time between weigh-ins and competition (typically 1–2 hours). Additionally, loss of weight at 1.5% of bodyweight per week to get down to the lowest allowable body fat percentage has allowed for weight loss during the season. However, this could lead to Relative Energy Deficiency Syndrome (RED-S). Research on this phenomenon is warranted. The normal person is about 60% water with ~67% being in the intracellular space and ~23% being in the extracellular space. The major ways to lose water at rest are ~60% through the urine, ~35% through losses in the sweat and lungs, and ~5% through feces. During exercise most of the water loss is through the sweat and lungs. Sweat rates are dependent on temperature, body size, and metabolic rate. As far as water intake ~60% is through fluids, ~30% comes from the foods we eat, and ~10% comes from metabolic reactions that produce water.

Amateur wrestling has a long history of rapid weight loss. This dangerous practice came to light in December 1997 when three collegiate wrestlers died due to rapid weight loss practices. One died of cardiac arrest while trying to lose 6 pounds while riding an exercise bike. The second died of heat stroke while riding a stationary bicycle and attempting to lose 4.5 lbs. The third died of kidney failure and malfunction of the heart wearing a rubber suit in a 92°F room (Litsky 1998). Clearly, 6 lbs is not that much weight and either is 4.5 lbs. Either those athletes were already quite dehydrated and/or another factor was involved in their death. One possibility that was discussed at the time of their deaths was the ingestion of ephedrine containing energy drinks. Clearly, the practice of severe dehydration is dangerous in the face of potent stimulants such as ephedrine containing energy drinks. This is because of the possibility of a cardiac arrhythmia and also the potential of the athlete to push the body past the point of normal defense mechanism, which would result in heat related illness such as heat exhaustion and fatigue prior to the possibility of death. However, the potential for cardiac arrhythmia (and cardiac arrest) is much less in individuals who are not naïve to stimulants such as ephedrine or caffeine. It would appear that the third wrestler who died because of kidney failure was severely dehydrated because kidney failure during dehydration occurs when there is lack of blood flow to the kidneys due to lack of plasma volume. This manifestation would clearly be facilitated by a 92°F room. Although tragic, there is a silver lining in these deaths. One, Senator John McCain proposed and passed through Congress, a legislation that resulted in the criminalization of ephedrine. Two, in 1998 the NCAA adopted new rules for weight control and management in their wrestlers. This and high-school practices to make the sport safer will be detailed in the following paragraphs. It must be noted that there is no hydration testing, body composition testing, or minimum weight for the Olympic Styles of Amateur Wrestling, i.e., International Wrestling (Men's Freestyle, Men's Greco-Roman, and Women's Freestyle).

HYDRATION TESTING

The first step in the Collegiate or High-School Folkstyle events is a hydration test. This is done by instructing the wrestler to come to the hydration testing session well hydrated. The wrestler then urinates and in college has had a urine specific gravity of no more than 1.020 (Gibbs et al. 2009) and in high-school (State of Ohio Wrestling Handbook) less than 1.025 (*OHSAA Wrestling Weight Certification Assessor's Handbook*). This tests for hypertonic hypohydration. That is dehydration occurs through sweating, as sweat is more dilute than the fluid inside the body, and therefore the plasma and urine become more concentrated than sweat and more concentrated than normal. Clearly a weakness in this Urine Specific Gravity Testing is the potential for the use of diuretics. With diuretics concentrated solute is lost in the urine with the water portion of the urine and the specific gravity of the urine stays the same or possibly becomes less leading to isotonic hypohydration or hypotonic hypohydration as opposed to hypertonic hypohydration. One suggestion is drug testing for commonly used diuretics in the urine used to measure specific gravity.

BODY COMPOSITION TESTING

Once the student-athlete "passes" the Hydration Test, he or she is ready for body composition testing. Usually, this is done by way of body density and specifically with skin fold calipers and appropriate equations for wrestlers (age and gender dependent) to calculate body fat % and fat-free mass %. At the high-school level, if the student-athlete/parent is not satisfied with the result they can retest body composition with hydrostatic weighing (underwater weighing) or whole body plethysmography (Bod-Pod). The lowest acceptable body fat in high school is 7% for boys and 12% for girls. In college the lowest acceptable body fat for men is 5%. After this "Alpha-Test" an athlete can lose 1.5% of bodyweight per week until they reach the lowest weight class where they would be closest to the lowest acceptable body fat (*OHSAA Handbook* 2018-2019; Gibbs et al. 2009).

BANNED PRACTICES

In the NCAA, prohibited practices are "rubber suits", saunas, steam rooms, hot boxes, laxative use, emetic use, diuretic use, excessive food and fluid restriction, wrestling room temperatures higher than 80°F, vomiting, and any artificial means of rehydration such as intravenous fluid administration (Gibbs et al. 2009). It appears that the only means for "losing the weight" is exercise and a sound diet. Clearly, this is a very good way to prevent the potential for health problems related to dehydration. Of note, however, the risk of in Sport (RED-S) still exists as a result of the allowance to lose 1.5% of bodyweight per week until the calculated desired body fat is reached. Research on this phenomenon is warranted.

WEIGH-IN TIMES

In the NCAA, weigh-ins before dual meets are one hour prior to dual meet competition and two hours prior to tournaments with one hour prior to tournaments on subsequent days. These weigh-in times have had an important effect on "weight-cutting" as rehydration time and recovery time are minimal before the match. In Olympic Style Wrestling at the Senior level there are 2 hours between weigh-ins and competition (Tim Pierson, Head UWW Official, Personal Communication). Additionally, there are one pound weight allowances after the first day at the NCAA tournament, i.e., a 125 lbs wrestler would be 125 lbs on Day 1, 126 lbs on Day 2, and 127 lbs on Day 3 (Nick Mancini, NCAA All-American Wrestler, personal communication). For United World Wrestling (UWW) competitions there is no weight allowance for most competitions from Day 1 to Day 2 of the two day tournaments. For World Cup and International Tournaments there is a 2 kg weight allowance for Day 2.

BODY WATER POOLS

For the 70 kg male (154 lbs) the total amount of body water is ~60% of bodyweight or ~42 kgs. The intracellular space contains the most water at about ~67% of total body water or ~28 kg. The extracellular space contains about ~23% of total body water at ~14 kg. The extracellular space can be further broken down into the intravascular space (fluid in the blood vessels and lymph vessels) and the interstitial space. Plasma volume is typically 3.5 L or 3.5 kg or ~8.3% of total body water and therefore represents the intravascular space while 14.8% or 6.2 kg are in the interstitial space or the space between cells. It must be remembered that a kg of water or sweat is equal to a L of water or sweat (Table 18.1).

TABLE 18.1
Body Water Compartments for Reference Man (70 kg Young Male)

	TBW	ICW	ECW	IVW	ISW
Liters	~42 L	~28 L	~14 L	~3.5	~10.5 L
%	100	~67	~33	~8	~25

TBW = total body water, ICW = intracellular water, ECW = extracellular water, IVW = intravascular water, ISW = interstitial water (Wilmore and Costill 1994).

It must be noted that when one sweats the fluid is first lost from the interstitial space, intravascular space, and then the intracellular space (Costill 1977).

WATER LOSS AT REST

Water balance is the balance between water output and water intake. Typically, we are in water balance, that is, the amount of water losses equals the amount of water gain. At rest, about 60% of the water output is by the kidneys and lost as urine. About 35% is lost through insensible loss through the lungs and sweat and another 5% is lost through the feces (Wilmore and Costill 1994).

WATER LOSS DURING EXERCISE

During exercise the majority of water loss is through evaporation of sweat and somewhat through respiration (insensible loss). This is dependent on (1) environmental temperature; (2) body size; and (3) metabolic rate. That is, the greater the environmental temperature the greater the rate of losses, the greater the body size the greater that rate of losses, and the harder the athlete is working the greater the sweat rate and loss through the lungs. Sweat rates in untrained athletes are approximately: 1 L/hour, while in trained athletes they can reach 1.5–2.8 L/hour (Costill 1977) in the heat. As you may expect these high sweat rates in highly trained athletes in the heat can lead to dehydration or body water deficits as it is impossible to drink enough fluid during these conditions that produce these high sweat rates. According to Wilmore and Costill (1974) during a marathon which lasts 2:15–6 hours for most individuals body water deficits of 6%–10% can be incurred despite efforts to replace fluid during exercise. A body water deficit of 2%, i.e., 2% dehydration can impair exercise performance (Armstrong et al. 1985). So, the question arises: Is fluid replacement important for optimal practice performance? The answer is a resounding yes with most wrestling practices lasting at least 2 hours.

DEHYDRATION AND PERFORMANCE OF INTENSE AND PROLONGED EXERCISE

WATER INTAKE

Roughly, 60% of our water intake is through fluids we ingest and about 30% comes from the foods we eat. Metabolic water, the water resulting from metabolic reactions in our body, provides the other 10% of water intake.

KEY POINTS

1. Rapid weight loss is generally ergolytic (impairs work performance) and has the potential to be life threatening.
2. The High-School Athletic Associations and the NCAA have instituted weight management rules that govern weight control in high school and the NCAA.

3. Weight management initiatives have been hydration testing, body fat testing, and reducing the time between weigh-ins and wrestling competitions.
4. Additionally, the loss of 1.5% bodyweight per week to get down to the lowest allowable body fat and weight is in practice but is of questionable benefit due to the existence of RED Syndrome.

19 Optimizing Physiology and Body Composition; Determining the Optimal Weight Category

Dehydration (by 2% of bodyweight) does not impair maximal effort brief exercise but does impair 6–7 minute effort power output. Food (energy) restriction will impair high-intensity exercise performance such as that performed during a wrestling match. Refeeding after weigh-ins would not appear to be sufficient to restore performance to that of the fed level in people who have fasted 24 hours or longer. Severe energy restriction would appear to affect hormones that are important to growth and recovery in adolescents. Periods of energy restriction followed by binge eating do not appear to have long-term effects on metabolism. Severe dehydration and energy restriction are not trivial with respect to health concerns as a number of wrestlers have died from such practices.

Rapid weight loss is defined as dehydration and/or energy (calorie or kilojoule) restriction in the few days prior to the match or tournament. With regard to the discussion of rapid weight loss, I will first discuss considerations regarding performance on the mat as this is typically the motivation for the rapid weight loss, i.e., they will be stronger at a lower weight class; although some individuals engage in rapid weight loss to "make the line-up". Second, I will discuss potential health related problems associated with dehydration and extreme exercise to lose weight as well as potential problems related to extreme energy restriction.

PERFORMANCE CONSIDERATIONS

It is common practice for high-school and collegiate wrestlers to undergo rapid weight loss. This rapid weight loss typically involves 1–3 days of dehydration, fluid restriction, and drastically reduced calorie (energy) intake. While this practice may seem advantageous for making the strength relative to bodyweight ratio optimal (and it is), rarely when competition is most important such as during the semifinals or finals of district, state, or national tournaments, when two opponents are evenly matched does the wrestling bout end in a pin (fall) fast (less than 30 seconds) or technical fall prior to the end of regulation time. *Wrestling Physical Performance*, as opposed to *technique*, during a bout in which two people are evenly matched is dependent on BOTH *the maximal strength/bodyweight ratio (Maximal Power Output)* and the ability to su stain a high power output to produce strength or power throughout *the whole*

6–7-minute match (Entire Match Wrestling Power Output). Research also shows that a wrestler needs to eat sufficient carbohydrate *and* be adequately hydrated to fuel *optimal wrestling physical performance* for the entire 6–7 minutes or more. This cannot be done when severely restricting energy (almost always carbohydrate energy) and fluid intake. Also, research shows that when a person is fasting (not eating or drinking calories) the muscle protein synthesis rate is not maximal compared to the fed state (Lambert et al. unpublished observations). In addition to these factors, there is sufficient evidence to suggest that there is a severe reduction in hormones in the blood which are essential for hormonal changes for growth and development and the potential recovery and maintenance of muscle mass of adolescent wrestlers when rapid weight loss is being undertaken (Roemmich and Sinning 1987a,b). The goal of amateur wrestling should be to *build character and promote the will to win by improving physical performance and maintaining health over the course of the season*, and these two goals can be attained under safe conditions. If one considers the potential drop in performance during practice and matches, as a result of rapid weight loss, as well as the potential effects of dehydration and food restriction on performance in the classroom, rapid weight loss is clearly counterproductive. A more prudent approach, although it requires more self-discipline, would be to lose body fat prior to the competitive season and to eat and drink correctly for optimal performance during training during practice sessions so that physical performance improves over the course of the season with the best performance occurring at the conference, state, and/or national tournaments.

EFFECTS OF DEHYDRATION ON MAXIMAL STRENGTH, POWER, FATIGABILITY, AND MUSCULAR ENDURANCE

EFFECTS OF DEHYDRATION ON MAXIMAL STRENGTH AND POWER

Relevance: Maximal strength and power are very important components of wrestling, for example during a single upper body throw attempt or during one attempted single leg or double leg shot. To summarize, moderate dehydration has little if any effect on maximal strength or power. Maximal strength or power may actually improve when expressed relative to the dehydrated body weight, that is the power/bodyweight or strength/bodyweight (Watson et al. 2005; Gutierrez et al. 2003; Cheuvront et al. 2006) Take-Home Message: From a performance perspective, if the match only lasts a few seconds then starting the match dehydrated would be alright. However, do not count on the match lasting only a few seconds and do not substantially dehydrate. A review of the studies cited for these findings can be found in Lambert and Jones (2010).

EFFECTS OF DEHYDRATION ON SHORT-TERM MUSCULAR ENDURANCE, FATIGABILITY, AND VO₂MAX

Relevance: The duration of exercise referred to below is generally speaking 30 seconds or greater to the end of 6 or 7 minute match. Therefore, this section is more important than the section immediately preceding this one. To summarize, moderate dehydration will result in an impairment of muscular endurance and lead to increased fatigability in muscular tasks that last longer than ~30 seconds, and the longer the event the more pronounced the premature fatigue at a given level of dehydration (Caterisano et al. 1988; Bigard et al. 2001; Caldwell, Ahonen, and Nousiamen 1984; Saltin 1964; Montain et al. 1998; Armstrong, Costill, and Fink 1985). A review of these findings can be found in Lambert and Jones 2010. Take-Home Message: If you start the match dehydrated and the match lasts longer than a few seconds your performance will be impaired. This clearly could be of greater magnitude if coupled with energy (usually carbohydrate) restriction.

EFFECTS OF ENERGY (CALORIE) RESTRICTION ON PERFORMANCE

FASTING EFFECTS ON HIGH-INTENSITY EXERCISE PERFORMANCE AND EFFECTS OF REFEEDING AFTER A FAST

In a physiological study that is very relevant to wrestling albeit during cycling exercise in recreationally active non-wrestlers, Gleeson, Greenhaff and Maughan (1988) compared the effects of a 24 hour fast to eating a normal meal, with the last meal being 4 hours prior to exercise, on time to fatigue at 100% of VO_2max. These investigators found that the 24 hour fast resulted in a 12.8% reduction in exercise time to fatigue compared with the normal diet treatment. The duration of exercise on the normal diet treatment was 243 seconds or roughly 4 minutes. This duration and intensity of exercise are very relevant to amateur wrestling as the average intensity of an amateur wrestling match is 95%–100% of VO_2max (See Lambert and Jones 2010; for an explanation). Thus, a 24 hour fast, which is relatively common practice for a wrestler, is very detrimental to high-intensity exercise performance like wrestling. The mechanism of action for this impairment in performance is not apparent and could be a reduction in brain glycogen (Matsui, Soya, and Soya 2019) as a 24 hour fast should not reduce muscle glycogen concentrations, as liver glycogen is the major source of blood glucose during a 24 hour fast. Muscle does not contain a phosphatase enzyme to release much glucose into the blood. Additionally, extracellular acidosis does not appear to be the cause of fatigue as when sodium bicarbonate was given after fasting 24 hour to reduce the acidosis performance was reduced to a similar extent as when a placebo was ingested (Lambert et al. unpublished observations). In a similar study of lower intensity and longer duration exercise, this same research group (Maughan and Gleeson 1988) had study participants fast for 36 hours and compared this long duration fast to a 10–12 hour overnight fast. In another arm of the study they had subjects fast for 36 hours but re-fed them with glucose (The simplest form of sugar, that is the form present in blood; 1 g/kg) 45 minutes prior to exercise. They found that the 36 hour fast reduced exercise performance (time to fatigue at a moderate intensity; 70% of VO_2max) by 35% and even with refeeding 45 minutes prior to exercise with a moderate amount of glucose the performance was still reduced by 22.7%. **The lesson from this study is that the highly detrimental effects of a prolonged fast cannot be reversed by refeeding 45 minutes prior to the exercise task.** This has profound implications for wrestlers as from a physiological standpoint a 35% reduction and even a 22.7% reduction (in the re-fed state) in wrestling physical performance is dramatic. Additionally, it is difficult to quantify differences in physiology, but a large difference in physical performance such as ~22.7%–35% reduction or elevation in exercise endurance by this much could be a great equalizer between a mediocre wrestler and a very good wrestler or poor wrestler and a mediocre wrestler in any venue. Thus, fasting would appear to be a detrimental practice for the competitive wrestler.

EFFECTS OF FASTING ON PROTEIN METABOLISM

In addition to the negative effects of fasting on exercise performance, fasting also causes muscle protein breakdown compared to the fed state (Fryburg et al. 1990). Fryburg et al. (1990) found that a 60 hour fast resulted in an increase in proteolysis with no decrease in protein synthesis. This proteolysis was illustrated by a 2–3 fold increase in the release of phenylalanine and leucine from the human forearm and a relatively high protein intake of 1.2 g/kg/day. Thus, a person can potentially lose hard earned muscle tissue by fasting. Indeed, one could speculate that you might see a reduction in muscle mass over the course of the season, by way of fasting on several occasions (i.e., prior to each match and tournament) over the course of the season. Clearly, this negative effect on muscle mass is not a situation that would augment wrestling performance.

Friedlander et al. (2005) reported that a 40% reduction in energy intake over 3 weeks reduced resting metabolic rate from 1,898 to 1,670 kcal/day. Protein was held at 1.2 g/kg/day well above the recommended daily allowance (RDA). There was a reduction in arm flexion performance but no decrease in aerobic performance. Nitrogen balance was negative throughout the study suggesting a loss of body protein with the 40% caloric restriction. Thus, it is important not to reduce your calories (energy intake) too much while losing weight. A gradual approach of losing no more than 2–3 lbs per week should be used (USA Wrestling Coach's Guide to Excellence 2005) during the weight loss phase of the year.

McMurray, Proctor, and Wilson (1991) reported that a caloric deficit to 92 kJ/kg fat-free weight/day (~1,500 kcal/day) resulted in no effect on run time at 85% of VO_2 max when high or normal carbohydrate diets were ingested but a decrease in total (−7%) and average (−6%) power output was observed when the Wingate Anaerobic test was undertaken under condition of a normal diet compared to the high-carbohydrate diet. Thus, the higher intensity task was affected but not the lower intensity task. Horswill et al. (1990) found similar results in college wrestlers (Table 19.1).

HORMONAL CHANGES

Roemmich and Sinning (1987a,b) performed two studies on weight loss and wrestling training and their effects on growth related hormones, physical characteristics, and physical performance. They found that a season of wrestling in 15–16 year old boys in which they were only taking in 24.7 kcal/kg/day or about 1,729 kcal/day for the 70 kg (154 lbs) wrestler, resulted in a decrease in insulin like growth factor-1 (IGF-1), free testosterone, total testosterone, and increase in cortisol and growth hormone, and an increase in sex hormone binding globulin (SHBG). Clearly, the decrease in IGF-1, increase in cortisol, decrease in free, and total testosterone are believed to be catabolic to skeletal muscle which is not what a wrestler or coach would want. Additionally, IGF-I is involved in long bone growth such as the humerus

TABLE 19.1
Fluid and Energy Restriction Pros and Cons

Restriction	Pros	Cons
Fluid intake and maximal power	Dehydration has little effect on maximal power output and would improve the power output to bodyweight ratio	Wrestling is not just maximal power output
Fluid intake and entire match wrestling power output	This would improve the maximal power output to bodyweight ratio.	Dehydration has been shown to impair exercise performance in events of similar duration and longer than a wrestling match
Severe (>39%) energy (calorie) restriction	None	Restricting carbohydrates has been shown to impair high-intensity exercise performance of a similar duration as a wrestling match
Fasting	None	Restricting carbohydrates has been shown to impair high-intensity exercise performance of a similar duration as a wrestling match

and femur. I believe this is due to an inadequate energy (calorie) intake relative to energy expenditure. *1,729 kcals is a low energy intake relative to energy needs of a wrestler of 154 lbs.* We have calculated the energy needs of a 70 kg, 5′ 7″, 16 year old wrestler at 3,286 kcals using the Harris Benedict Formula (Harris and Benedict 1918), specific dynamic action at about 10% of energy needs, and 650 kcal/hour for a 2 hour wrestling practice. It appears that this extreme energy restriction (a ~47% reduction below energy needs) is likely causing the hormonal problems seen in the studies of Roemmich and Sinning (1987a,b). An associated problem noted by Friedlander et al. (2005) with a 40% reduction in energy intake is a 12% reduction in resting metabolic rate or the ability to combust energy at rest. The diet in the studies of Roemmich and Sinning (1987a,b) was 61% carbohydrate 24% fat, and 15% protein. That would put the protein intake at 65 g which is at 0.93 g/kg/day. This is above the RDA. This further supports the role of a low energy intake and not inadequate protein intake in the alterations in the hormones/growth factors measured by Roemmich and Sinning (1987a,b) and the reduction in resting metabolic rate seen by Friedlander et al. (2005). Again, it is important to eat adequate calories during the season as you should try to be weight stable and fuel your training sessions during the season. Additionally, eating adequate protein will hasten recovery (see below). The condition of the athletes in the older studies of Roemmich and Sinning (1987a,b) may fall under the umbrella of the condition of Reduced Energy Deficit in Sport (RED-S) as tagged recently by the International Olympic Committee (IOC) and their position stand (2018).

HEALTH CONSIDERATIONS

The death of three previously healthy collegiate wrestlers from November 7th–December 9th, 1997 as a result of rapid weight loss practices brought into light the potentially life threatening nature of "weight-cutting" as practiced in US amateur wrestling. So, more importantly than not being advantageous to optimal wrestling performance, rapid weight loss has the potential to be life threatening to you if you are a wrestler or to your wrestlers if you are a coach. Regardless of the amount of weight lost there are potential risks. First, there are possibly genetic factors that make one individual more susceptible to dehydration/heat illness than another. Thus, because of these genetic factors, some individuals may have problems at lower levels of dehydration and/or lower levels of hyperthermia (increased environmental and hence body temperature) than others. Another factor that comes into play regarding a wrestler's ability to tolerate exercise in the heat is that the level of heat acclimatization. This simply means how adapted is the individual to exercise in the heat. Adaptation comes from repeated exposures to the heat and exercising in the heat over the course of days and weeks. Thus, at the beginning of the season or when it is a wrestler's first time trying to make a given weight, they may be more susceptible to problems related to the heat and dehydration than later in the season.

What kind of problems does severe dehydration cause? Dehydration can cause problems with mood and cognition (the ability to think), delirium, and headache (Popkin, D'Aaci, and Rosenberg 2010). Additionally, dehydration can result in a reduction in blood volume which will increase heart rate, and if the reduction in blood volume is great enough there will be a reduction in blood pressure (Popkin, D'Aaci, and Rosenberg 2010). Along with this reduction in blood pressure is a reduced blood flow to the kidneys that if severe enough can cause renal ischemia (Popkin, D'Aaci, and Rosenberg 2010). This is simply a reduction in blood flow to the kidneys. No blood flow and no oxygen delivery, no oxygen delivery and tissues can only work for a very short time without oxygen. Eventually, portions of the tissue, in this case the kidney, could die as a result of the lack of oxygen resulting in an infarction. We all know what a myocardial infarction is, a heart attack. Thus, tissue dying off such as kidney tissue will impair the function of that organ. Clearly, not a situation a teenager or young adult wants.

Exercise related problems associated with dehydration are numerous. When a person exercises in a normal room temperature environment the muscles require blood flow for oxygen delivery for aerobic muscle contraction and to remove things like carbon dioxide and lactic acid (Guyton and Hall 2006). Additionally, blood flow goes to the skin to dissipate heat to the external environment. As the temperature increases, for example when a wrestler wears a sweatshirt, blood flow increases to the skin, so there becomes this competition between the skin and the working muscle for blood flow. A wrestler only has so much blood volume to go around. What happens when you dehydrate? You have even less blood volume to go around because that is where a large portion of the fluid is lost from the blood. So your muscle and skin need blood flow but blood volume is reduced through dehydration. In the dehydrated state, blood flow to the skin is reduced as the muscle wins in the competition for blood flow. As blood flow to the skin is reduced, heat storage in the body increases.

Thus, the body's internal temperature goes up. This increases the rate at which you sweat. Obviously, this leads to a greater level of dehydration if the goal is to lose weight through dehydration and you are not replacing the lost fluid. Eventually if you lose enough fluid from the blood through exercise as heat, there will be insufficient blood volume to perfuse the heart musculature (through the coronary arteries) and you could go into cardiac arrest. Also, it is possible that this cardiac arrest is caused by an electrolyte imbalance from extreme dehydration; this can lead to arrhythmias (altered heart beats) and cardiac arrest (Guyton and Hall 2006). Regardless of the exact mechanism, in all three of the cases where the collegiate wrestlers died in 1997, they had gone into cardio-respiratory arrest. The bottom line: exercise in the heat (this can mean wearing warm clothing) and dehydration can cause wrestlers to die. Therefore, weight loss through energy restriction (caloric restriction) and *gradual weight loss* (2–3 lbs per week) prior to the competitive season rather than *rapid weight loss* (i.e., fasting, severe calorie restriction, and extreme dehydration) is the way to protect the safety of wrestlers of all age levels.

EFFECTS OF A WRESTLING SEASON INVOLVING ENERGY RESTRICTION ON RESTING METABOLISM

In two separate studies performed by Dr. Chris Melby and co-workers (Schmidt et al. 1993), one in which wrestlers were studied over 2 years and one in which wrestlers were studied over 3 years, it was shown that in weight cycling wrestlers: those wrestlers that continually lost weight and regained it over the course of the season, *did not have a reduction in resting metabolic rate or in other words they did not get fat over time by reduced resting energy expenditure*. In other words, the weight cycling did not reduce their ability to burn calories at rest. This is contrary to the popular notion that there is a reduction in the resting metabolic rate as a result of continual weight cycling and a spontaneous weight gain without eating more in years after the athletes' competitive career. Other possible explanations as to why former wrestlers appear to gain more weight over the course of their lifetime than their non-wrestling counterparts likely deal with the energy intake side (i.e., eating more than they expend) of the energy balance equation (as the resting metabolic rate deals with the energy expenditure side of the equation). In other words, for psychological reasons and/or possibly reasons related to appetite, former wrestlers may eat more calories than their non-wrestling counterparts over the course of their lifetime (especially after they are done wrestling). It is possible that this may require counselling and education on proper eating behaviors.

KEY POINTS

1. From a performance standpoint, dehydration of about 2% of bodyweight does not impair maximal instantaneous power or strength but will impair muscular endurance. Therefore, since muscular endurance is in an important attribute for a wrestler, dehydration should not be undertaken if you want to optimize performance.

2. Severe dehydration could be life threatening. So if you can find a way to beat the Alpha Test, it is not in your best health interest to do so.
3. Although fasting impairs high-intensity and endurance exercise performance, the mechanism remains elusive but may be brain glycogen depletion. Also fasting impairs muscle protein synthesis which is not in the best interest of the wrestler wishing to optimize body composition.
4. The 40%–50% energy restriction observed in some studies have led to reduced resting metabolic rate and reduced anabolic/growth hormone/factor concentrations.

20 The Case against Rapid Weight Loss

Energy balance is the balance between energy (caloric) intake and energy output or caloric expenditure. Energy intake is simply the energy that you ingest. Energy expenditure is broken down into resting energy expenditure, energy expenditure related to exercise, that related to the digestion, absorption, and metabolism of food, and non-exercise induced thermogenesis such as fidgeting. Weight loss for amateur wrestling should happen before the season while during the season weight should be maintained and practices and matches fueled with optimal nutrition for performance and recovery. I have come to the conclusion that successful weight loss can be boiled down into taking four components into consideration: (1) Documenting Energy Intake; (2) Monitoring Bodyweight; (3) Monitoring Muscular Strength; and (4) Calculating Resting Metabolic Rate and estimating the amount of energy to ingest (Calories). The prudent goal is a loss of 1–2 lbs/week over the course of the weight loss period since energy or caloric restriction of 40% or greater can reduce resting metabolic rate and cause negative hormonal changes. During the pre-season weight loss phase athletes should take in adequate protein for heavy weight training and long-distance running and should ingest 60% CHO, 20% Protein, and 20% Fat. Twenty percent protein will allow for ~1.5 g Protein/kg bodyweight/day. Diets with about this much more protein or higher protein should spare fat-free mass (i.e., muscle mass) from being lost as a result of weight loss.

Despite what the Diet Gurus say *weight loss* is quite simple: A Calorie is a Calorie! It is like an old "balance" type of scale with energy intake on one side and energy output on the other side. Although *weight loss* is not *easy* it is quite *simple: simply take in less calories than you burn.* This is what is meant by the term Negative Energy Balance. *However, the composition of the weight loss (fat or muscle) is affected by the composition of energy intake, i.e., a diet that is higher in protein than normal will preserve muscle mass when losing weight.*

ENERGY BALANCE

When one is in energy balance the amount of calories or kilojoules they are taking in is equal to the amount of calories they are expending. When one is in *negative energy balance* the amount of calories or kilojoules they are taking in is less than the amount they are burning and they are losing weight. When one is in *positive energy balance* the amount of calories they are taking in is more than they are burning and they are gaining weight. Although the composition of the weight lost (i.e., whether it is muscle or fat) will vary based on a number of things, **weight loss is that simple**: Eat less calories than you need.

ENERGY INTAKE

This is the amount of calories you take in (calorie intake).

CALORIE INTAKE

A gram of protein has 4 calories when burned in a flame based device (in a device called bomb calorimeter) while that of carbohydrate also has 4 calories and fat has 9 calories. However, there is an extremely important difference in the calories of these macronutrients when taken in the body. This will be discussed next.

ENERGY OUTPUT

Exercise and movement of all forms, energy expended to digest food, and resting metabolism.

FOUR COMPONENTS OF ENERGY EXPENDITURE

1. Resting metabolism

   Resting metabolism or the calories we burn when we are totally inactive are to a very large extent determined by our bodyweight. In fact just by knowing a person's bodyweight, the resting metabolic rate can be determined with great accuracy. *Resting metabolism is the largest component of energy output* unless you are performing an Iron Man Competition or performing a marathon or longer events which are not an everyday occurrence (roughly 100 kcal/mile walking or running). An established estimate of resting energy expenditure is given by the Harris–Benedict Formula (Harris and Benedict 1918). For men the equation is

$$\text{Resting Energy Expenditure} = 66.4730 + \left(13.7516 \times \text{weight}\,(\text{kg})\right)$$

$$+ \left(5.0033 \times \text{height}\,(\text{cm})\right) - \left(6.7550 \times \text{age}\,(\text{yrs})\right)$$

   For women the equation is

$$\text{Resting Energy Expenditure} = 655.0955 + \left(9.5634 \times \text{weight}\,(\text{kg})\right)$$

$$+ \left(1.84965 \times \text{height}\,(\text{cm}) - 4.6756 \times \text{age}\,(\text{yrs})\right)$$

So for the 90 kg male who is 6′ 0″ tall and is 16 years old, the resting energy expenditure would be 2,111 kcal/day.

   Another way to calculate and get similar results is to take 1 Metabolic Equivalent (MET; 3.5 mL/kg/min), convert this into calories expended, and you multiply each liter of oxygen consumed by 5 (5 kcals/L of oxygen consumed). So if someone weighed 90 kg it would be 3.5 mL/kg/min × 90 kg × 24 hours/day × 60 min/hour = 435,600 mL of oxygen (435.6 L) consumed per 24 hours × 5 kcals/L of oxygen consumed = 435.6 L × 5 kcal/L = 2,178 kcals/day. These value represents an approximation of the amount of calories burned at rest over the course of a day for a 90 kg or 198.4 lbs person.

2. Thermic Effect of Food (Specific Dynamic Action)

The thermic effect of feeding (specific dynamic action) makes up approximately 10%–15% of energy expenditure. That is the digestion, absorption, and storage of food and drink. The majority of available data suggest that there is an increased energy expenditure associated with the ingestion of protein (digestion, absorption, storage), and this leads to satiety also known as appetite suppression (Westererp et al. 2004).

3. Exercise

Clearly exercise is quantitatively the most important way to *expend* calories when trying to shed fat weight. The most important factor with regard to burning calories during exercise is just that…burning calories during exercise. The harder and longer you work, the more calories you burn, period. You burn more calories the harder you train: five calories per liter of oxygen consumed: the harder you work the more oxygen you consume and the more calories you burn. So, relatively brief intense workouts are advantageous if caloric expenditure is important. If more calories need to be expended then longer intense workouts fit the bill. There is one caveat here for the wrestler. The harder you work, the more muscle glycogen you use (Gollnick et al. 1973). This glycogen is extremely important for high-intensity efforts like wrestling. Therefore, when trying to lose or *maintain weight during the season*, in addition to the intense workouts you undergo, long *slow*-distance exercise walking, slow running, and stationary cycling will burn calories (primarily fat), spare muscle glycogen, and reduce the conversion of fast fibers to slower fibers for practices and matches. However, it is my contention that you should lose weight before the season, *maintain weight during the season*, and fuel practices and matches with a large amount of carbohydrate, fluid, and adequate protein while in energy balance (not losing or gaining weight) during the season. You can also use a tape measure around the waist at the umbilicus (belly button) to track progress. Clearly, to optimize physique, in addition to losing fat, you need to gain muscle in the pre-season. This should be done by resistance training (weight training) with relatively heavy weights to optimize strength gains, accordingly some muscle mass gains will come with this. Ideally, the male wrestler would want to come in at 7% body fat the lower limit for high-school wrestlers (5% for the college wrestler) and 12% body fat for female wrestlers. The idea would then be to maintain optimal body composition throughout the season by matching energy output (mainly exercise) with energy intake (caloric intake).

NON-EXERCISE ACTIVITY (NEAT)

This for the active athlete is a relatively small amount of calories but for a sedentary person is a fair amount of calories. Basically this encompasses things like fidgeting and movement that is not considered exercise. For our purposes this is negligible.

Nutrition for wrestling should be approached from a general framework. First you should lose fat prior to the season as, extra fat will not help you, and this portion of wrestling should be taken care of *prior to the competitive season in the pre-season*. At the same time you should attempt to maintain your muscle strength that you have developed over the previous months in the off-season and pre-season during the competitive season. During the season, *after you have lost the fat*, you should concentrate on eating to fuel your workouts as wrestling practices involve very high energy expenditures and carbohydrate use and maintaining your strength which means a high-carbohydrate diet (8–10 g/kg/day) and eat about two times the Recommended Daily Allowance (RDA) of Protein 1.5 g/kg/day (RDA is 0.8 g/kg/day). Prior to tournaments a wrestler should eat a high-carbohydrate diet or glycogen load because wrestling uses glycogen **at *rate*** (use per unit time) **faster** than a long-distance runner. When you eat a very high-carbohydrate diet prior to a tournament you have enough carbohydrate available for four matches; eat less carbohydrate and fatigue is likely to occur prior to the end of the fourth match (Lambert and Jones 2010).

A STRATEGY FOR OPTIMAL PERFORMANCE BY WAY OF FAT LOSS IN THE PRE-SEASON

Fat loss, as noted above, is important for the wrestler, as generally speaking State and National Rules suggest that 7% body fat is deemed a safe level for the health of boys. Fat loss prior to the season is best achieved by energy restriction and aerobic exercise. When restricting your energy the most important thing to remember is that a calorie is a calorie. You need to concentrate on gradual loss of weight over time, and this is the most important factor for maintaining muscle strength/muscle mass and it will also maintain your immune system health. Energy restriction or calorie restriction should be used for the means to lose fat or to change one half of the energy balance equation. As a general guideline you should lose is 2–3 lbs a week but no more (USA Wrestling Coaches Guide to Excellence 2005). Actually, 1–2 lbs per week is more desirable as it will require less energy/calorie restriction. The amount of fat loss should be dictated by body fat testing as prescribed by State and National Athletic Association rules as these have been formulated for wrestler safety.

Aerobic exercise should be used as the means to lose fat on the energy expenditure side of the energy balance equation. Aerobic exercise is activity such as running 1–5 miles. The advantage to long-distance running is that in addition to being very good for fat loss it improves your maximal oxygen consumption; the single best measure of physical fitness, and an important factor in your wrestling success. Additionally, the fact that you can sustain it for long periods of time allows you to burn many calories without overstressing your body. When lifting to maintain muscle strength during this time if your strength declines you may be overdoing the energy restriction or running and may want to increase your calories or decrease your running or both.

OPTIMAL WEIGHT LOSS PRIOR TO THE SEASON

It is my opinion (based on research; see "Positive Benefits of Wrestling" chapter), personal experience as a high-school wrestler, and 37 years of studying Exercise Physiology and Nutrition that most of the weight loss occurring in amateur wrestling should occur prior to the competitive season and should be almost entirely body fat loss rather than through dehydration and fluid and food restriction. As will be discussed in a subsequent section, from the standpoint of optimal performance, if weigh-ins are 1 hour before wrestling you should not dehydrate more than by about 1.5% (~2.2 lbs, 1 kg, or 1 L) and if weigh-ins are 2 hours prior to wrestling you should not dehydrate by more than 3.0% (~4.4 lbs, 2 kg, or 2 L). These values are based on maximal rates of fluid emptying from the stomach, and hence a reasonable measure of rehydration of about 1 L/hour. To preserve muscle mass a person probably should not undergo more than a 3 lbs weight loss per week. Logically, a 2 lbs weight loss or even a 1 lbs weight loss per week will preserve fat-free mass (muscle mass) better than more drastic weight loss. As discussed above in the Energy Balance Section: To lose ~1 pound a week you must be in a *negative energy balance* of ~500 calories/day (3,500 kcals/week; a combined deficit at the present weight from energy restriction and/or exercise as 3,500 kcals is 1 lbs of fat). To lose ~2 pounds a week from your present weight you must be in a negative energy balance of ~1,000 calories/day (7,000 kcals/week) and to lose ~3 pounds a week you need to be in a negative energy balance of ~1,500 calories/day (10,500 kcals/week).

A FOUR COMPONENT METHOD FOR WEIGHT LOSS

From my experience in my own training and in Exercise Physiology teaching and research of ~37 years I have come to the conclusion that successful weight loss can be boiled down into taking four components into consideration: (1) Documenting Energy Intake; (2) Documenting Bodyweight; (3) Documenting Muscular Strength; and (4) Calculating Resting Metabolic Rate and estimating the amount of energy to ingest (Calories). The goal is a loss of 1–2 lbs/week over the course of the weight loss period.

1. Energy (Calories) Ingested
   The most important component in weight loss is the calories ingested and calories expended. Although the different macronutrients (Carbohydrate, Protein, and Fat) are important for performance and muscle mass, it is the caloric balance (Calories In vs. Calorie Out) that determines weight loss or gain. You must take in less calories than you eat to lose weight and to gain weight you must take in more calories than you expend. For caloric intake for weight loss part of the equation, counting calories is extremely important. I would suggest buying a book with all of the calories of known foods in it. These are relatively inexpensive. What gets measured gets managed.
2. Bodyweight
   Another important component of the weight loss program is knowing your bodyweight. Bodyweight encompasses the sum total of energy consumed

and energy expended and therefore is a very powerful measurement. By knowing your bodyweight and your caloric intake, an exact determination of your total caloric expenditure is not extremely important, and maintaining muscle strength would appear to be an important way to make sure one is not restricting energy intake too much and exercising too much. This is a good thing because measuring total energy expenditure is quite difficult. A suitable surrogate for bodyweight is waist circumference (measured at the belly button (umbilicus) with a tape measure).

3. Muscular Strength

Monitoring muscular strength is extremely important when losing weight for three reasons: (1) Monitoring strength is very important when training to see where your strength is going over the course of a season, (2) Monitoring your strength is a very good way to see if you are restricting your energy intake (calories or kilojoules) too much, and (3) Monitoring your strength is a very good way to determine whether the training load during pre-season workouts is too high. Clearly, discerning between #2 and #3 above is quite difficult but for the purpose of physical performance is irrelevant. Simply use muscle strength as your guide to assess performance/ nutritional status (i.e., overtraining and undereating) over the course of the season. Choose three exercises and monitor your strength before weight loss for some period of time. Lose weight and keep a close watch on the strength of these three lifts. I would suggest Bench Press, Back Squat, and Dead Lift or some other form of systematic strength assessment using exercises relevant to wrestling. If you lose weight too fast and/or your training load is too high you will lose too much strength. At the least you should attempt to maintain strength on these three lifts while losing body fat. Because you do not monitor fat-free mass with hydrostatic (underwater weighing), skin fold calipers, bod pod (whole body plethysmography), etc. on a routine basis these strength exercises will be your "check" on muscle mass/muscle strength.

4. Calculating Resting Metabolic Rate and Estimation of Calories to Ingest

Using the resting metabolic rate calculation from above (3.5 mL/kg bodyweight/min; ACSM 2014 or the Harris–Benedict Formula (1918)), allowing for genetic differences in resting metabolic rate, taking into consideration differences in physical activity level the ACSM resting metabolic rate calculation (ACSM 2014; 3.5 mL oxygen/kg bodyweight/min × 60 min/ hour × 24 hours/day × 5 kcal/L oxygen consumed) can be used as a rough estimate of required calories to maintain bodyweight. Again, remember it is for **RESTING** metabolic rate. Thus, the more physical activity one does the further from the truth will be this estimation (Resting Metabolic Rate) of how many calories you should be eating. Generally speaking, the careful wrestler will want to start to monitor his caloric intake prior to the season to the start of wrestling practices to determine the calories to maintain bodyweight when not training extensively. This can be done easily by monitoring bodyweight before and after 7 days and monitoring caloric intake daily for those 7 days. In this way, the wrestler will have a feel for how many calories it takes to maintain bodyweight without the extensive energy expenditure associated with wrestling practices. However, by monitoring bodyweight, muscle strength, and caloric intake the wrestler can closely monitor his own progress. Clearly, a primary determinant of a promising wrestler's performance is his/her chosen weight class in conjunction with his/her nutritional practices. Not eating enough carbohydrate/calories on a daily basis during training at a low weight class is worse than choosing a higher weight class and eating properly. The calculation for estimating energy expenditure and therefore how many calories to ingest = resting metabolic rate (RMR) (Harris–Benedict Formula + Specific Dynamic Action (10%–15% of daily energy expenditure) + Exercise Energy Expenditure.

A REASONABLE STRATEGY FOR FAT LOSS

Cutting carbohydrates is a strategy many people use to lose weight. This is not in the best interest of the active athlete. Additionally, the reason cutting carbohydrates works is because of the decrease in calories ingested and also loss of water weight as each gram of glycogen stores 3–4 grams of water. This effect can also be achieved by a low-fat diet with less performance decreasing effects than a low-carbohydrate diet. Also, a diet without carbohydrate is not only not advantageous to exercise but it is in fact dangerous and counterproductive (hypoglycemia during driving, taking a test, practice, etc.) as the brain's main choice of fuel is glucose (Guyton and Hall 2006). The amount of carbohydrate required for *certain amounts and intensities* of exercise is still under debate. Also, this carries over to optimal brain function and performance in the classroom. Therefore, why not error on the conservative side when involved in intense exercise such as wrestling. Therefore, restricting carbohydrates is not a preferred way to lose weight as athletes need carbohydrates to train and students need carbohydrate to think. Again, a calorie is a calorie and you have a balance sheet less calories in than you need and you lose weight more calories in than you need and you gain weight. Not to say adequate amounts of protein, carbohydrate, and fat are not important. *Again, what I am saying is that optimal weight should be attained before the season and you should provide sufficient carbohydrate for training, studying, and performing the activities of daily living when you are losing weight.* The emphasis of wrestling training should be to improve your physical performance over the course of the season. This cannot be done on a carbohydrate deficient diet. Therefore, low or no carbohydrate diets should be discouraged when dieting or training high-school and college athletes as a calorie is a calorie in fat loss and carbohydrates are required for adequate and optimal functioning during intense exercise. For the fat loss portion of the year (pre-season) I would suggest a diet that is 60% carbohydrate, 20% protein (**this should keep your protein at least 1.5 g/kg bodyweight/day**) and 20% fat. Again, eat less calories than you need. First assess your energy needs by a 7-day dietary recall where you write down everything you eat for 7 days (without a weight change) use your calorie counting book and determine the calories in each food/meal/day and then calculate an *average* caloric intake per day over the 7 days. Weight loss should be 1–3 lbs per week. A one pound loss of fat may be achieved by reducing your calories by 500 per day over the course of a week.

For example, if you need 3,000 kcal eat 2,500 kcal for a week as you will lose water with the fat. When weight loss ceases then reduce your kcals again by 500 kcal/day. You may want to use a tape measure and waist circumference (at the umbilicus) for determining abdominal fat loss. You will need more carbohydrates the more active you are in the pre-season. In the subsequent section, I will describe research in which dietary protein is elevated in a weight loss diet while not being devoid of carbohydrates and muscle mass was retained very well and where fat loss was high. For sample menus, see USA Wrestling Coaches Guide to Excellence available with a Bronze Coaching Certification (pp. 169–170). To reiterate a 7-day dietary recall should be performed to get an average calorie intake per day and then drop your calories by 500 kcal so if the average for the week is 3000 kcals drop to 2500 kcals/day. Ingest a 60% carbohydrate, 20% protein, and a 20% fat diet. This will provide you with enough carbohydrate to train and at least 1.5 g/kg of protein to maintain muscle mass when losing weight.

The Amount of Muscle and Fat You Lose during Dieting Will Depend on the Amount of Protein You Eat If you want to hang on to your fat-free mass (muscle mass) to a greater extent, research suggests that a higher protein diet amount *while dieting* is advantageous. Layman et al. (2009) performed a study in which study subjects reduced their calories by 500 kcal/day while eating 1.6 g of protein/kg/day and less than 170 g of CHO/day and compared this to those individuals reducing their calories by 500 kcal/day and eating 0.8 g protein and greater than 220 g CHO/day at 4 months those on the high protein group lost 22% more fat mass than those on the low protein intervention. No difference in weight loss occurred. Thus, the high protein group held onto more fat-free mass. Thus, eating about 2× (1.5 g/kg bodyweight) the RDA of protein (0.8 g/kg bodyweight = RDA) will substantially preserve fat-free mass (muscle mass) when dieting. It must be emphasized that these research subjects were not exercising so in this instance the low-carbohydrate intake is o.k. In addition, there is a relevant study in resistance trained athletes from Dr. Kevin Tipton's group in Birmingham, England (Mettler et al. 2010). These investigators had younger men (~25 years of age) reducing their caloric intake to 60% (control group went from 3,443 cals/day to 2066 cals/day; a relatively large amount of energy restriction). One group ate 2.3 g/kg bodyweight of protein (roughly 2.9× the RDA) and the other group ate 1.0 g/kg bodyweight of protein. These investigators reported that the group that ate 1.0 g/kg protein/day lost roughly 5.3 times more fat-free mass (for our purposes muscle mass) than the group that ate 2.3 g/kg bodyweight of protein per day. The fat-free mass loss for the high-protein group was 0.3 kg, whereas that for the low-protein group was 1.6 kg. Thus, **when losing weight (not to be confused with training for competition)** with the intent of losing body fat and not muscle mass a higher protein diet at the expense of carbohydrates in the diet is the way to go (Table 20.1).

The Amount of Muscle You Lose during Dieting Will Depend on the Degree of Energy Restriction

Lose weight slowly if you don't want to lose muscle. A rate of weight loss of 2–3 lbs per week is commonly believed to be safe and effective. Losing weight slowly and in

TABLE 20.1
Selected Weight Reduction Diets

	Description	Pros	Cons
Low calorie	Reduced energy intake, primarily fat reduction	Weight loss is good usually if counting calories and gradually reducing them	Hunger present and protein not adequate usually to maintain fat-free mass
Low carbohydrate	Reduced energy intake, carbohydrate restriction (~50 g/day)	Weight loss is good usually if carbohydrate is restricted	Too low in carbohydrate for live wrestling training
Mediterranean	High fiber, high unsaturated fat, low protein	A heart healthy effective weight loss strategy without documenting energy intake would greatly facilitate ease of use	May be too low in protein to retain fat-free mass during weight loss and no documentation, i.e., inexact
High protein moderate carbohydrate	High protein (~2.0 g/kg bodyweight/day) at least 130 g of carbohydrate/day	Excellent for retention of lean body mass during energy restriction	May be too low in carbohydrates for live wrestling training and other forms of exercise

the pre-season makes sense and is safer, leading to better performance in the classroom, on the mat during practice, and during matches.

KEY POINTS

1. Energy Balance = Energy Intake compared to Energy Expended.
2. While Energy Intake is simply what you eat, Energy Expenditure follows a Four Component Model: (1) Resting Metabolic Rate, (2) Exercise Expenditures, (3) the Thermic Effect of Feeding, (3) Non-Exercising Activity (NEAT; negligible). Calories to Ingest = Resting metabolic rate (Harris–Benedict Formula) + Specific Dynamic Action (10%–15% of energy intake) + Exercise Induced Energy Expenditure.
3. Weight loss should be before the season and should consist of a Long Slow-Distance Aerobic Exercise and a low-calorie (60% CHO, 20% Pro, 20% Fat), high-protein diet. Start slow with a −500 kcal change and be gradual.
4. Useful weight loss tools are (1) Energy (Calories) Ingested; (2) Bodyweight; (3) Muscular Strength; and (4) Calculating Resting Metabolic Rate and Estimation of Calories to Ingest.

21 Optimal Nutrition for Maintenance of Body Composition and for Fueling Training during the Season

The optimal in-season diet for maintaining body composition attained during the pre-season and for fueling and recovering from training sessions would appear to have 8–10 g/kg body weight of carbohydrate, 1.5 g/kg bodyweight of protein, and 0.7 g/kg of bodyweight of fat. Pre-practice nutrition should consist of 70–250 g of carbohydrate, while during practices fluid should be ingested at the rate of ~1 L/hour, and contain ~50 g of carbohydrate and contain electrolytes. Post-practice nutrition should contain 1.5 g/kg body weight of high-glycemic index carbohydrate (first hour; 1.2 g/kg/h thereafter) and at least 20–40 g of high- quality protein. Low- fat chocolate milk is an excellent choice.

GOALS OF NUTRITION FOR TRAINING DURING THE SEASON

The two *major goals* of your overall nutrition program for training during the season are as follows: (1) To provide adequate carbohydrate for training sessions and hydration to fuel training sessions and (2) to provide adequate carbohydrate, protein, and fluids to recover from training sessions to become ready for the next training session. *Because training is the most important aspect of your match success.*

With regard to Goal 1, the overall goal of your training from a physiological standpoint is to improve the maximal sustainable power output for 6–7-minutes or more of a match. Improvement of maximal *absolute* power production (explosiveness) is best left to the pre-season (strength training) and you should try to maintain this level of maximal power production during the season. To improve the maximal sustainable power output during the 6–7-minute match you need to "build the engine" through optimal conditioning, but equally important, you need to "fuel the engine" with proper nutrition, primarily carbohydrate nutrition. Clearly, you need to eat properly prior to training properly. So "fuel the engine", train very hard but very smart by pushing the limits of your maximal sustainable power output in practice, and then repeat with each practice. Thus, eating optimally, and training hard, your maximal sustainable power output will increase. The end result is that you will have a very high horse power engine when you go for 6 or 7 minutes. Research supporting my contention that proper training and carbohydrate nutrition can improve overall power output over time is provided by the work of Simonsen et al. (1991) in rowers. These individuals had rowers train intensely for 4 weeks and provided 10 g of carbohydrate/kilogram of bodyweight/day compared with a control group who ate 5 g of carbohydrate/kilogram of bodyweight/day. The group that ate 10 g of carbohydrate/kilogram of bodyweight per day improved their performance by 4% over the 4 week period. This is a large amount of carbohydrate, and you probably need a concentrated carbohydrate liquid to accomplish this or to eat some other form of simple sugars such as sugary cereals or chocolate milk in high amounts. I would suggest 2× strength Gatorade or Powerade (powder form). A high-carbohydrate diet during intense exercise has recently been supported by the work of Stellingwerf, Maughan, and Burke (2011). Additionally, the question remains: what is the improvement over the course of a *full season* (and not just one month) when eating adequate carbohydrate and training intensely. Many wrestlers, in my opinion based on available data from research studies, have stunted their performance by eating inadequate amounts of carbohydrate as a result of cutting weight, not optimally fueling their training sessions, and not being able to train as hard as they may have. This ultimately leads to a leveling off or a decline in the maximal sustainable power output during the 6 or 7 minute match. I will talk about maintaining adequate hydration and post-exercise carbohydrate and protein nutrition in subsequent sections.

OVERALL COMPOSITION OF THE DIET

If things have gone as planned, prior to the season, you have reduced your body fat down to a relatively low percentage without losing too much muscle mass. The goal now is to keep it there and eat to fuel and recover from workouts as well as prepare for competition. Based on our previous discussion, at this stage stay on about 8–10 g of carbohydrate/kg of bodyweight, 1.5 g of protein/kg of bodyweight, and 0.7 g of fat/kg of bodyweight. An example would be a 70 kg wrestler (154 lbs). Using these amounts of carbohydrate, protein, and fat he/she would be taking 630 g of carbohydrate, 105 g of protein, and 49 g of fat. This ends up being 3,381 kcals. This would appear to be an optimal number of calories given a resting metabolic rate of 1,764 kcals (ACSM calculations 2014) and assuming ~60 minutes of wrestling @ 100% of VO_2max (VO_2 max ~60 ml/kg/min; pretty typical of wrestlers) in a 2 hour practice (~1,260 kcals). Given the thermic effect of feeding being 10% of kcals ingested caloric requirements would be ~332.4 kcals and your caloric intake would be ~3,324. Thus, energy needs and energy intake would be pretty well matched. However, the recommendations to stay out of Relative Energy Deficiency-Syndrome (RED-S) in which energy intake minus the energy cost of exercise should be 45 kcal/kg Fat Free Mass/day (IOC Position Stand on RED-S 2018) suggest an energy intake of 4,500 kcals given the information on the practice above and 70 kg wrestler @ 7% body fat. If you need to increase the calories to stay in weight maintenance, keep the ratio 60% carbohydrates, 20% protein, and 20% fat and increase total calories appropriately. To assess if this is the right amount of calories for weight maintenance, keep your training at a steady rate (if a coach is reading this it is probably possible to do this as a team) for a week, calculate how many calories you are consuming daily, and titer

TABLE 21.1
Overall Dietary Breakdown for Optimal In-Season Performance

Macronutrient	Amount to Ingest	Percent of Total Energy Intake
Carbohydrates	~8–10 g/kg bodyweight/day	~60
Protein	~1.5 g/kg bodyweight/day	~20
Fat	~0.7 g/kg bodyweight/day	~20

your calories to maintain bodyweight. *In other words, if you are losing weight or waist circumference throughout the week then eat more calories, if you are gaining weight or waist circumference, eat less.* This will give you a good idea of how many calories you need to maintain your weight. Your body does not like to use protein (more correctly amino acids) for energy when it is in energy balance but does when you are in **negative energy balance** (i.e., losing weight). The actual grams/kg you take in is more important than the percentages as follows. Your carbohydrate intake should be roughly 8–10 g/kg/day and you should eat more carbohydrate if you are running out of energy during the day and less carbohydrate when you have had short or easy workouts. Protein (~1.5 g/kg/day) and fat (0.7g/kg of fat/day) should stay constant but you should titer or alter your carbohydrate intake relative to your needs as described above, more carbohydrate during or before days of intense training and less carbohydrate during easy days or less intense workouts. Remember carbohydrates spare protein (Bowtell et al. 2000). Thus carbohydrates are oxidized and protein left behind to do its job which is rebuilding or building muscle (Table 21.1).

PRE-AND DURING PRACTICE NUTRITION

Eat your pre-practice meal 1–4 hours prior to practice and make it primarily carbohydrate. Eat 70–250 g of carbohydrate. Again, make sure you are staying on ~8–10 g/kg carbohydrate/day, 1.5 g of protein/day, and ~0.7g of fat/day. So for three meals for a 70 kg person: 233 g of carbohydrate for breakfast, 233 g for lunch, and 233 g for dinner. Again, this carbohydrate ingestion may impair fat oxidation, but fat oxidation is of minimal importance during intense exercise such as wrestling (Little et al. 2009).

Adequate carbohydrate and fluid ingestion *during practices* is rarely addressed by coaches or wrestlers. This is unfortunate as dehydration and lack of carbohydrate ingestion during training sessions will have deleterious effects on performance and wouldn't it be great to perform at your best and improve every practice? In a study relatively relevant to wrestling from the standpoint of the duration of exercise reflecting the duration of practice is a study by Below et al. (1995) from Dr. Coyle's laboratory at the University of Texas. These investigators found that drinking a large volume of fluid during intense exercise of 1 hour in duration was far superior (6.5% improvement) than drinking a small volume of fluid or drinking no fluid. Additionally, these investigators found that taking in adequate carbohydrate was far superior to taking in no carbohydrate during this 1 hour of exercise (6.3% improvement). Finally, these investigators found that ingesting both fluid and carbohydrate during 1 hour of intense exercise was far superior to ingesting either of the two during 1 hour of exercise. *The bottom line is that ingesting fluid and carbohydrate during intense training sessions such as a wrestling practice will substantially improve performance during that session.* What is our goal? To improve the maximal sustainable power output during the 6 or 7 minute match and possibly an overtime match. Thus, ingesting adequate fluid and carbohydrate will allow you to train hard enough to induce adaptations in the cardiovascular and muscular systems and improve your power output over the course of a match, multiple matches during one day, and during multiple-day tournaments such as state tournaments for high-school athletes and the NCAA tournament for collegians. So what are the guidelines? To maintain carbohydrate supply to working muscles during a practice, the guidelines are to take in 30–60 g of easily digestible carbohydrate per hour (ACSM Position Stand on Exercise and Fluid Replacement 2007; Sawka et al. 2007). With regard to fluid intake, one should maintain bodyweight or attempt to during practice. I would suggest that the lighter wrestlers replace what they lost with 500 mL/h, the middleweights replace with 1000 mL/h, and the heavyweights replace with 1,500 mL/h with a carbohydrate–electrolyte solution as this is reflective of sweat rates (replace what you sweat out). Most studies have shown the best results with regard to hydration and optimal carbohydrate delivery with a ~6% carbohydrate–electrolyte solution such as Gatorade or Powerade. This will provide both adequate fluid and adequate carbohydrate to fuel optimal performance during practice.

POST-PRACTICE NUTRITION

The goals for post-practice nutrition are to rehydrate, restore muscle glycogen stores back to optimal levels, and to provide adequate protein to repair and potentially build muscle. These goals are aimed at recovery for the next training session! With regard to restoring muscle glycogen and increasing the synthesis of muscle proteins: TIMING IS EVERYTHING! It is important to eat protein and carbohydrate about **30 MINUTES AFTER EXERCISING** (Kersick et al. 2008). The reasons for this are as follows: (1) the muscle is sensitive to the effects of insulin and there is an insulin-like effect of exercise and (2) and muscle blood flow is still adequate for amino acid and carbohydrate delivery to the muscle for uptake. With regard to ingesting fluid it is important to restore hydration levels back to the pre-practice level. What is not universally known is that this in most cases requires ingesting a fairly high amount of sodium with your fluid (addressed in the post-weigh in the Rehydration section).

CARBOHYDRATE

It is important for optimal muscle glycogen restoration to eat 1.5 grams of easily digestible carbohydrate/kilogram of bodyweight in the first 30 minutes after exercise to stimulate the maximal rate of muscle glycogen restoration (Kersick et al. 2008). With regard to what type of carbohydrate to eat, the available data would suggest eating high-glycemic index carbohydrates in the first 30 minutes after exercise. In reality, taking in a high-glycemic index carbohydrate diet all the time would probably promote high glycogen concentrations all of the time as a result of the dramatic increase in insulin. *However, this type of diet if eaten every day and is the major source of carbohydrates may have long-term negative health implications, and therefore it is not recommended in the off-season when energy expenditure and therefore carbohydrate oxidation is low, i.e., titer energy intake to energy needs.* However, taking in a bolus (1.5 g/kg bodyweight) of high-glycemic index carbohydrate in the first 30 minutes after exercise will maximize the rate of muscle glycogen restoration as a result of high insulin concentrations. With this in mind, I would suggest taking in high-glycemic index carbohydrates in the first 30 minutes after exercise. The majority of carbohydrate consumption during the remainder of the day should be low-glycemic index carbohydrates such as whole grains. If you have trouble reaching the goal of 8–10 g of CHO/kg/day intake of carbohydrates with low-glycemic index carbohydrates, then top your stores off with a high-glycemic index carbohydrates during the day to reach the goal as these are typically more concentrated/lower volume sources and therefore take up less room in the gastrointestinal tract and therefore you will feel less full. See glycemic index of selected foods in the table at the end of this book.

PROTEIN

With regard to the timing, amount, and type of protein, it has been shown that eating protein immediately after exercise is superior to than waiting 2 hours with regard to promoting muscle building (Andersen et al. 2005). With regard to the type of protein, whey protein has benefits other than the fact that it is anabolic, such as anti-oxidant properties (Ha and Zemel 2003). The amount of protein should be between 20 and 40 g (Kersick et al. 2008). Antioxidants may stave off muscle fatigue (Reid 2016) by neutralizing free radicals produced during intense exercise as these free radicals have been implicated in fatigue during intense exercise. Another property of whey protein is that it is a protein that breaks down fast and causes a rapid increase in protein synthesis. Casein is a protein that breaks down slowly but is as effective in stimulating protein synthesis as whey (Tipton et al. 2004). To obtain 20 g of protein from milk a person would have to drink 2.5 cups or 20 ounces of milk. I would suggest skim milk. Better yet, to get both the post-exercise protein and carbohydrate requirement low-fat chocolate milk is a very good choice. One cup of low-fat chocolate milk has 8 g of protein, and 30 g of carbohydrate of which 28 g are sugar. Sugar (high-glycemic carbohydrate) is very good post-practice. So, you need approximately 20–40 g of protein post-practice and 1.5 g of carbohydrate per kg bodyweight for the first 30 minutes post-exercise (Kersick 2008; 1.2 g/kg/h). Thus, for the 70 kg wrestler (reference man; 154 lbs) he or she should drink 3.75 cups of low-fat chocolate milk within 30 minutes of the end of the workout. This would be equivalent to 30 ounces of low-fat chocolate milk (to get the appropriate amount of sugar and protein) for the 154 lbs wrestler. Because this relationship is a direct relationship a coach could determine how much low-fat chocolate milk that a person should drink by the following equation:

$$30 \text{ ounces}/154 \text{ lbs} = x \text{ ounces/wrestlers weight (lbs)}$$

So you would put in a given wrestlers weight in the bottom right side of the equation, and solve the equation for X (ounces), to find out how much low-fat chocolate milk a wrestler should drink in the 30 minutes after a wrestling practice.

With regard to the type of protein: whey or casein, which is better? To reiterate, Tipton et al. (2004) found that the ingestion of casein and whey were similar in the net positive muscle protein balance they caused after resistance exercise. Thus, whey or casein should be consumed after resistance exercise. Again, do not forget to ingest your 1.5 g of protein/kg bodyweight/day.

REHYDRATION: FLUID AND SODIUM

Rehydration is dictated by the sodium content of the ingested fluid and the volume of the fluid ingested (Mitchell et al. 2000; Sharp 2006). Additionally, the fluid ingested must have some carbohydrate for sodium and glucose co-transport in the small intestine (Jeukendrup et al. 2009). Additionally, the greater the volume of the fluid in the stomach the greater the gastric emptying rate (Costill and Saltin 1974) due to the effects of hydrostatic pressure. So from the standpoint of sodium and glucose, water does not do the job. Drink 150% of what you lost due to dehydration (Mitchell et al. 2000; Sawka et al. 2007) and make sure there is adequate sodium in the beverage such as Gatorade, Powerade, or Pedialyte. The sodium will allow you to retain the fluid in your system by losing less in the urine. Additionally, all Gatorade, Powerade, and Pedialyte have adequate amounts of sodium for glucose–sodium co-transport in the small intestine. Gatorade and Powerade are better for glycogen restoration and Pedialyte is better for rehydration based on their respective carbohydrate and sodium contents.

KEY POINTS

1. The two *major goals* of your overall nutrition program for training during the season are as follows: (1) To provide adequate carbohydrate for training sessions and hydration to fuel training sessions and (2) to provide adequate carbohydrate, protein, and fluids to recover from training sessions to become ready for the next training session.
2. A high-carbohydrate diet (8–10 g/kg bodyweight) is important to maintain high-intensity exercise capacity, especially when practices can last two hours or more. Remember, this is about the equivalent of a marathon running race.
3. Eat 70–250 g of carbohydrate 1–4 hours before practice to optimize practice exercise performance.
4. Carbohydrates and fluids independently improve exercise performance, and their combined effects are approximately double of either one alone: drink a carbohydrate–electrolyte solution during practice.

5. Try to begin to restore carbohydrate and protein stores within 30 minutes of practice rather than wait. Research shows 30 minutes is better than waiting 2 hours.
6. For rehydration after practices drink 150% of the fluid volume lost (what you lost in kg plus 50%; a kg is equal to a L) of carbohydrate–electrolyte solution. Chocolate milk is an excellent post-exercise fluid, carbohydrate, and protein restoration fluid.

22 Nutrition for a Single Match, a One-Day Tournament, and a Multiple-Day Tournament

BACKGROUND

The maximal gastric emptying rate is about 1 L/h or 2.2 lbs/h, less for energy dense solutions such as chocolate milk. This should be taken into consideration when one is rehydrating from dehydration. Additionally, there is only enough stored muscle glycogen for 4.3 collegiate matches in a high-glycogen state. Thus, it is prudent to eat a high-carbohydrate diet (8–10 g/kg CHO/day) at all times during the season. Additionally, eating foods with high sodium concentration during the season will help to maintain hydration status. Prior to major events, it would appear important for the wrestler to eat a high-carbohydrate diet and reduce his/her activity level for 3 days prior to the event to maximize muscle glycogen concentrations.

FLUID REPLACEMENT

The background or basis regarding fluid replacement for a single match, single-day tournament, or multiple-day tournament is quite simple: If you step on the mat with your bodyweight 2%–3% below your normally hydrated weight you will fatigue early while wrestling at your optimal intensity or you will have to decrease your optimal intensity, neither of which leads to optimal performance. Thus, either do not dehydrate to make weight or dehydrate by a manageable and legal amount so that when you step on the mat you are not dehydrated by greater or equal to a 2% reduction in bodyweight from your normally hydrated weight. Using the guidelines for rehydration post-weigh in is the way to go to maximize the rate of rehydration after weigh-ins. However, if the extent of dehydration is too great, getting the body's fluid balance back to a range where performance is optimal is impossible given the time limitations and the limitations imposed by the wrestler's gastrointestinal tract (maximal gastric emptying rates of 1 L/h).

1. Carbohydrate Intake
   We need to account for the post-exercise oxygen consumption (calorie burning) and the fact that many times, during anaerobic exercise, muscle glycogen is broken down to muscle lactic acid, and this source of

carbohydrate (lactic acid) does not get oxidized but gets converted back to glucose in the liver (by a process known as gluconeogenesis). With regard to post-exercise calorie burning I have some data in which we evaluated the time to fatigue at 100% of VO_2max and how it differs between genders. What is interesting from this data is that we kept the exercise participants on the mouthpiece and nose clip for 15 minutes after they reached the point of fatigue. Now this exercise results in fatigue in roughly 4–6 minutes, and the energy for such exercise to fatigue is derived from ~50% anaerobic metabolism and ~50% from aerobic metabolism. Due to the fact that a large portion of the energy for this exercise is derived from anaerobic metabolism, this must be paid back after exercise and is done so by caloric expenditure after exercise termed the Excess Post-Exercise Oxygen Consumption (EPOC). Just picking out one male subject data, we see that there is considerable caloric expenditure after exercise. This subjects' time to fatigue at 100% of VO_2peak was 4 minute and 15 seconds. During exercise this subject burned 54 calories nearly all of which were carbohydrate (13.5 g). During the 15 minutes after exercise, the subject burned 51 calories all of which were carbohydrate (12.75 g). This really shows that the calculation of caloric expenditure *during* intense exercise with a high-anaerobic component is only part of the picture regarding caloric expenditure resulting from this type of exercise. Again, as far as the total grams of carbohydrate oxidized (burned up) this is not an astronomical amount. However, we only followed the subjects out for 15 minutes after exercise, and at this time the calories expended were still 100% carbohydrate calories and 0% fat calories.

2. In addition to the post-exercise oxygen consumption, calorie expenditure, and carbohydrate combustion, if intense exercise is undertaken for longer than a few seconds (5–6 seconds; Wilmore and Costill 1994) lactic acid production from glycogen is a requirement for the production of adenosine triphosphate (ATP) under anaerobic conditions (without oxygen availability) and/or conditions where there is a very high demand for ATP production over a short amount of time. Therefore, even if the muscle glycogen is not combusted to carbon dioxide and water but forms lactic acid, it is equally *essential* for the production of ATP. The metabolic product lactic acid is in essence a carbohydrate (2–3 carbon lactic acid molecules are produced from one 6 carbon glucose-6-phosphate molecule from glycogen). As such, lactic acid can be used to re-establish muscle carbohydrate stores. This is done by the conversion of lactic acid to glucose in the liver, the movement of glucose from liver to blood to muscle, and the building up of muscle glycogen from the glucose (Cori Cycle; Stryer 1988). You do not need the glycogen *any less* due to the fact it is not ultimately getting oxidized ... you need it regardless of whether it is getting oxidized (by oxygen to CO_2 and H_2O; aerobic conditions) because glycogen is going to lactic acid under anaerobic conditions to produce the essential energy source for muscle contraction: ATP. Thus, you don't actually combust all of the glycogen by oxidative metabolism but you break it down by anaerobic metabolism to lactic

acid which produces ATP for muscle contraction, and the lactic acid which reaches the blood from the muscle after the match can then be reconverted to glucose in the liver and be taken up by muscle to make glycogen. We also do not know how much glycogen you can count on remaking from the post-exercise blood lactic acid concentration. This means, although you can count on getting some glycogen restoration *during the recovery period* from the high blood lactic acid concentration generated *during the match,* we, as scientists, do not know how much glycogen restoration you can count on getting without eating after a wrestling match. As a result, to take the guess work out of this situation of: "how do I know how much fuel I have in the muscle after a match during a tournament" you should start with the carbohydrate maximized in the muscle (by eating 8–10 g of carbohydrate/ kilogram of bodyweight/day; Simonson et al. 1991) and continue to eat copious amounts of carbohydrate during the day of a tournament. Clearly, based on muscle biopsy data *under low-carbohydrate* conditions there is enough muscle glycogen for one match (Spencer and Katz 1991). Much of this glycogen is converted to lactic acid; without eating *we do not know how much of the blood lactic acid is converted back to glucose by the liver and to glycogen by the muscle.* If, under high muscle glycogen conditions, all of the muscle glycogen was oxidized, in other words, converted to CO_2 and water along with the production of ATP, *there would only be enough glycogen there for 4.3 high-school matches or 3.7 collegiate matches with high muscle glycogen concentrations* (Spencer and Katz 1991). It is probable that some of the lactic acid produced during each match during the day can be converted by the liver into glucose and glucose can be converted to glycogen in the muscle during the recovery period. How much? *We do not know. So it is a prudent practice for wrestlers to go into a tournament with their glycogen levels maximized and that they eat copious amounts of carbohydrate* (400–600 g; 8–10 g/kg of bodyweight) *during the* day, if they can for multiple-day tournaments. This probably should take the form of concentrated fluids double strength Gatorade or Powerade from powder and concentrated sugar containing candy, grape juice, sugary cereals, and low-fat chocolate milk (Tables 22.1 and 22.2).

FLUID REPLACEMENT DURING A SINGLE-DAY OR MULTIPLE-DAY TOURNAMENT

This is quite simple: follow the post-weigh-in guidelines in this book and to sum them up: drink to keep your bodyweight at your pre-dehydration level. This occurs by drinking enough fluids to maintain bodyweight and taking in enough sodium through food and fluids so that you retain the fluid that you ingest. One easy way to do this is by drinking a solution that is high in sodium (~50–100 mmol/L) or eating a low volume of something that is very salty (chicken noodle soup; ~180 mmol/L sodium) to cause water retention and stimulate further consumption of fluids. Again use bodyweight as the guide. Drink 150% of what you have lost to get back to normal bodyweight (Mitchell et al. 2000).

TABLE 22.1
Nutrition for a Single Match (Time Constraints: 1–2 h Post Weigh-In)

Wrestlers' Disposition	What to Drink and Eat	Purpose
Dehydrated without liver or muscle glycogen depletion	Drink a 5.5%–6% sports drink with electrolytes at 1.5× dehydration level	Rapid rehydration and provide adequate carbohydrate for match physiology
Dehydrated and glycogen depleted	Drink a 10% carbohydrate soln. at 1.5× weight loss: non-caffeinated Pop's or sodas come to mind or grape juice and eat two medium bananas	Relatively rapid rehydration (slower than with a sports drink) but provides adequate carbohydrate for glycogen restoration and potassium
Euhydrated and glycogen depleted	Eat sugary cereal and skim milk and grape juice @ 250–400 g carbohydrate in the 1–2 hours post-weigh-in grape juice	Restore glycogen in liver and muscle
Euhydrated, well rested, and well fed	Eat sugary cereal and skim milk and grape juice @ 7–250 g carbohydrate in the 1–2 hours post-weight-in grape juice	The ideal situation. You have eaten breakfast, and lunch, and you just need to top off the glycogen stores; ready to train the next day

TABLE 22.2
Nutrition for Multiple-Day Tournaments

Wrestlers Disposition	Plan for Optimal Nutrition Despite Little Time
Wrestling (2–5 matches in one day). Drink 5.5%–6.0% CHO sports drinks between matches for CHO and fluid needs. Low-fat chocolate milk will assist in meeting the CHO and protein requirements at the right column	8.0-10.0 g Carbonate (CHO)/kg bodyweight 1.5 g Protein (PRO)/kg bodyweight 0.7 g Fat/kg bodyweight Rehydrate at 1.5× bodyweight losses

CARBOHYDRATE NUTRITION IN THE DAYS PRECEDING ONE-DAY OR MULTIPLE-DAY TOURNAMENTS

Based on previous discussions in this book, it should be fairly obvious where this discussion is going. It is my contention, based on the available research data, that having the muscle and liver loaded with carbohydrate, is a very good idea prior to single-day or multiple-day tournaments. This being the case, you have to eat sufficient amounts of carbohydrate to increase the amount of glucose the muscle and liver are exposed to and therefore improve carbohydrate delivery and storage as liver and muscle glycogen. This is done by eating 8–10 g of carbohydrate/kilogram of bodyweight/day for 3 days before the competition (Glycogen Loading). On the carbohydrate expenditure side of the equation it is prudent for workouts to be low volume and low intensity for 3 days prior to the competition so that sufficient carbohydrate can be stored in the muscle, in other words, to decrease carbohydrate combustion or burning in the 3 days prior to the tournament. If you don't decrease the volume and intensity of workouts you will not *STORE* carbohydrate in the muscle as glycogen. *BOTH* of these conditions: A high-carbohydrate diet *AND* a reduction in training volume and intensity must be met for sufficient muscle glycogen storage. Additionally, some two day tournaments for high-school wrestlers now require the wrestlers to compete in five matches per day. Not only is the 3 days of reduced training volume and intensity important for glycogen storage but it is probably not a bad idea to back off training volume and intensity in the days leading up to the tournament in preparation for the extreme physical demands of ten matches in two days. This could be thought of as a mini-taper. Tapering, by its nature, allows the wrestler's physiology and psyche to recover and super-compensate in preparation for an impending extreme physiological and psychological challenge (Mujika 2009).

KEY POINTS

1. The maximal gastric emptying rate is about 1 L/h, or in other words 1 kg/h or 2.2 lbs/h. Keep this in mind when you have weigh-ins 1 hour prior to wrestling, i.e., it's best not to weigh in more than 2.2 lbs dehydrated.

2. *There is only enough glycogen in skeletal muscle for 4.3 high-school matches or 3.7 collegiate matches with high muscle glycogen concentrations.* Keep this in mind for practices and many match tournaments as well as multiple-day tournaments (i.e., eat 8–10 g CHO/kg of bodyweight/day).

3. To stay rehydrated, after matches, make sure you are taking in sufficient sodium. Chicken noodle soup is a great source of sodium, and therefore you will retain fluid and maintain plasma volume at optimal levels. Urine color is always usually a good indication that you are hydrated. Look for clear and not dark urine.

4. It is a prudent practice for 3 days before a multiple-day tournament to eat a high-carbohydrate diet and reduce practice intensity and duration, as both of these conditions must be met to store adequate glycogen in skeletal muscle. This would be a mini-taper.

23 What and How Should the Wrestler Eat Post-Weigh In?

Under conditions of relatively severe dehydration, solutions such as Pedialyte which has a high sodium content but is still hypotonic should be ingested, while during less severe dehydration sports drinks such as Gatorade or Powerade can be consumed. If dehydration is not a factor, hypertonic solutions such as chocolate milk which will augment muscle glycogen storage and muscle protein synthesis should be consumed. Grape juice can also be consumed as it has a very high glycemic index, but this should be done if you are worrying about carbohydrate storage as it is not a protein source.

After weighing in, there are approximately 1–2 hours prior to the start of competition. The maximal gastric emptying rate (rate at which fluids are emptied from the stomach) is ~1 L/h (1,000 mL/h). This is equivalent to 2.2 lbs. Therefore, if you dehydrate by more than 2.2 lbs (for 1 hour duration between weigh-ins and competition) or by 4.4 lbs (for 2 hour duration between weigh-ins and competition) you will not be able to go on the mat properly hydrated. So calculate what you have lost due to dehydration in lbs or kgs and drink a total of 150% of that volume (lbs or mL; drinking 150% of the volume ingested has been shown to be superior to drinking 100% of the volume lost for optimal rehydration; Mitchell et al. 2000) as you lose fluid through urination. Take the volume you have calculated and break it down into 2 feedings for 1 hour weigh-ins and 4 feedings for 2 hour weigh-ins. Start drinking immediately after you weigh-in (Table 23.1).

OPTIMAL POST WEIGH-IN REHYDRATION PLAN

EATING AND REHYDRATING AFTER WEIGHING IN WITH LOW-GLYCEMIC INDEX FOODS OR HIGH-GLYCEMIC INDEX FOODS AND DRINKS?

The glycemic index is an indicator of how fast different types of carbohydrates breakdown in the body and is different than the old simple vs. complex carbohydrate way of looking at things. High-glycemic index foods break down fast in the body and as such raise insulin levels relatively high. This is good for glycogen restoration as insulin pushes the glucose from the blood stream into the muscles and liver. In fact, Burke et al. (1993)s have shown that in the 24 hours post-exercise it is better to eat high-glycemic index foods and fluids than low-glycemic index foods and fluids for muscle glycogen restoration. This is all well and good for training or competition *the next day,* but one drawback of high-glycemic index food and fluid ingestion is

TABLE 23.1
Rehydration (and Carbohydrate Intake) Guidelines for Three Different Situations

1. Least desirable: If you have not been eating adequately during the few days prior to the match and have been exercising vigorously to lose weight via dehydration and caloric restriction your muscle glycogen stores are probably somewhat low. In this case drink a 6% carbohydrate–electrolyte solution (like Gatorade or Powerade) every 30 minutes in a volume that is 150% of the volume you are dehydrated by. This will supply both fluid and carbohydrate to the muscles and blood. The large volume ingested each time you drink it facilitates gastric emptying (Costill and Saltin 1974). Thus, the suggestion is drink 150% of what you lost at each time point so that when you are done drinking prior to wrestling you will have ingested 150% of that lost during dehydration. *In this case, it would be a good idea to take in a high-sodium food during the day as well so you can retain the fluid you ingested. When in the dehydrated or euhydrated state (normally hydrated) you do not have to worry about high blood pressure.*

2. Desirable if cutting weight: If you have been *eating properly (a high-carbohydrate diet)* and you have just moderately dehydrated the day before the match or tournament then a 3% carbohydrate solution with 60 mmol/L (Pedialyte is a better choice than a solution with a lower sodium concentration.) *This is the better way to lose weight immediately prior to a match or tournament if you are only losing a maximum of 4.4 lbs before a match or tournament where there is 2 hours from weigh-in to match or 2.2 lbs when match to weigh-in is 1 hour.* This is the case again because the upper limit for emptying fluid from the stomach is 4.4 lbs in 2 hours and 2.2 lbs in 1 hour. The higher sodium concentration will allow your body to retain the fluid better after you have ingested it. Like the previous example with the 6% carbohydrate–electrolyte solution, the 3% carbohydrate–electrolyte solution should be ingested in a volume of 12 ounces every 30 minutes beginning immediately after weigh-ins and ending 30 minutes prior to the beginning of wrestling. *It is unnecessary in this situation to take in a high-sodium food during the day since there is adequate sodium in the rehydration solution.*

3. Do not cut weight in the days and weeks prior to the match: Most desirable: Normally rehydrate after the previous evenings workout with a 6% carbohydrate–electrolyte solution and do the same after weigh-ins (use your pre-workout bodyweight as the guide regarding how much to rehydrate). Since you have been eating a high-carbohydrate diet for 3 days prior to the competition (8–10 g carbohydrate/kilogram bodyweight/day), backing off on the intensity and volume of workouts for the past 3 days, and you don't have to worry about restoring fluid balance, your muscles and liver are carbohydrate loaded with carbohydrate and your cardiovascular system and muscles are full of water prior to competition for maximum oxygen and nutrient delivery to the cells and removal of metabolic end-products that can impair muscle contraction. *You are ready to maintain the highest power output your cardiovascular and muscular systems can maintain for 6–7 minutes (Maximal Wrestling Match Power Output). This highest power output you can maintain over the 6–7 minutes is the result of the conditioning that has been undertaken and is your engine. This highest sustainable power output for 6–7 minutes as dictated by the size or horse power of your engine (which is determined by your ability to produce anaerobic and aerobic work) can only be attained if there is sufficient fuel in the gas tank (muscle glycogen) and if the carburetor (oxygen delivery) and exhaust system (carbon dioxide and lactic acid removal) are in optimal operating condition, and this is largely determined by the amount of fluid circulating in the cardiovascular system where oxygen, carbon dioxide, and lactic acid are dissolved. If there is insufficient fluid in the cardiovascular system oxygen delivery to working muscles will be impaired as will be the removal of carbon dioxide and lactic acid.*

that the high-insulin levels that accompany this type of carbohydrate ingestion can inhibit fat release from the fat cells and therefore fat use. Theoretically, this may raise insulin levels and inhibit fat oxidation during prolonged exercise. However, this situation does not closely mimic a wrestling match or matches in one day. In an another important study, Little et al. (2009) compared the ingestion of low- and high-glycemic index foods 3 hours prior to exercise on intermittent high-intensity running on a treadmill. This protocol was set up to mimic a soccer match. They found that the high-glycemic foods 3 hours before exercise did impair fat use during exercise, but no difference in exercise performance was observed between high- and low-glycemic index food ingestion. Both treatments improved performance to a similar extent compared to a fasting trial. Thus, the moral of the story is fat use is of limited importance *during very intense exercise*. Therefore, if something impairs fat use during high-intensity exercise, it is likely not a problem.

Suggestion: After weigh-ins consume high-glycemic index foods (a big bolus immediately after weighing in) equivalent to at least 1.5 g of carbohydrate/kilogram of bodyweight (Kersick et al. 2008)). This will improve performance during the tournament compared with eating low-glycemic index foods by way of glycogen storage. Also, this will help during more than one-day tournaments. This is because, as stated above, a high-glycemic index food ingestion is better than low-glycemic food ingestion for raising insulin levels and muscle glycogen restoration. Below is a glycemic index of different foods the closer to 100 the greater the glycemic index. A few obvious high-glycemic index foods for after weigh-ins are corn flakes, cheerios, jelly beans, and Gatorade. For a more comprehensive discussion of the glycemic index, see Foster-Powell, Holt, and Brand-Miller (2002). Below is the table of the glycemic index of selected foods with pure glucose being set as the standard at 100. Again, only eat high-glycemic index foods during the season when energy turnover (energy use and energy intake) are extremely high.

THE CASE FOR CHOCOLATE MILK

In the post-exercise period there is a need for three things, liver and muscle restoration, muscle protein synthesis, and rehydration. An excellent choice to serve all three purposes is chocolate milk. Chocolate milk is a rich source of complete protein and simple carbohydrate (high-glycemic index). Additionally, there is a high quantity of calories in chocolate milk which augments both glycogen restoration and muscle protein synthesis. An excellent study from John Ivy's group (Born et al. 2019) at the University of Texas suggests that chocolate milk is a beverage of great practical importance for the high-school athlete. In this study, these investigators pre- and post-strength tested (composite squat and bench press) high-school boys and girls with 5 weeks of strength and conditioning training between the pre- and post-test. After each session the groups either drank a carbohydrate supplement or chocolate milk. Upon post-testing the chocolate milk group had about a 12% increase in composite strength, while the carbohydrate group has a 2%–3% increase in strength. This was a statistically significant difference in strength gains. The chocolate milk provided 16 g of protein and 300 kcals while the carbohydrate supplement provided 0 g of protein and 160 kcals. Clearly, it would appear advantageous to drink chocolate milk in the immediate post-exercise period from a practical standpoint of strength gains. What is less important and less clear from a practical standpoint is was it the protein, the calories, or a combination of the two that lead to the improvements. Both drinks provided the same amount of carbohydrate, and although not assessed, endurance/fatigue testing may be assumed to be similar since the same amount of carbohydrate was provided. Regardless, chocolate milk, for a number of reasons, would appear to be a prudent choice for maximizing strength performance related to training in adolescents. Another positive benefit of chocolate milk is the osmolality of the beverage. Because of the protein in the chocolate milk as opposed to beverages without protein, the osmolality would be higher. This would lead to greater fluid retention and long-term rehydration. A caveat of drinking chocolate milk would be if rapid rehydration were of paramount importance as it empties from the stomach relatively slow. In this case, it would be prudent to drink something with lower osmolality and energy density such as Pedialyte. Water is ok, but since it lacks sufficient osmolality, it will "go right through you", i.e., a high urine volume would be expected leading to a long-term fluid retention. Also, the lack of sodium and glucose in water makes it slow to absorbed in small intestine relative to something like Pedialyte.

KEY POINTS

1. The maximal gastric emptying rate should be taken into consideration when thinking about rehydration: 1 L/h or 1 kg/h or 2.2 lbs/h.
2. If highly dehydrated (post-practice for example) one should drink Pedialyte as it is hypotonic and contains less carbohydrate and more sodium than water or regular "sports drinks".
3. If moderately dehydrated (like after a normal practice), a "sports drink" should be ingested as it is higher in carbohydrate and lower in sodium.
4. The best answer is to remain euhydrated (normally hydrated) as a result of drinking adequate amounts of fluid to maintain hydration. This is the best way to ensure that exercise performance is maintained at optimal levels.
5. With regard to eating high- or low-glycemic index food, eating high-glycemic index foods is advantageous from the standpoint of muscle glycogen restoration after exercise however, this practice should be limited to the competitive season as high-glycemic index carbohydrates and lack of exercise may be deleterious to glucose homeostasis (Table 23.2).

TABLE 23.2
Glycemic Index of Various Foods

Food Category

Breads

White bread	70
Wholemeal bread	69
Pumpernickel	41
Dark rye	76
Sourdough	57
Heavy mixed grain	30–45

Legumes

Lentils	28
Soybeans	18
Baked beans (canned)	48

Breakfast Cereals

Cornflakes	84
Rice bubbles	82
Cheerios	83
Puffed wheat	80
All bran	42
Porridge	46

Snack Foods

Mars bar	65
Jelly beans	80
Chocolate bar	49

Fruits

Apple	38
Orange	44
Peach	42
Banana	55
Watermelon	72

Dairy Foods

Milk, full fat	27
Milk, skim	32
Icecream, full fat	61
Yogurt, low fat, fruit	33

24 Dietary Supplement Use in Wrestlers

Protein supplements may stave off a protein deficiency in adolescent wrestlers as the protein requirements of resistance trained adults is 1.6 g/kg body weight per day, and youth and adult protein requirements are similar. Additionally, this may be the case since total energy intake was reportedly somewhere in the neighborhood of ~1,500 calories in adolescent wrestlers prior to the current weight loss regulations. Creatine monohydrate has been found to be effective in improving anaerobic exercise capacity (Greenhaff et al. 1993; Casey et al. 1996; Birch et al. 1994). Many youth athletes may already be using creatine monohydrate as an effective nutritional ergogenic aid. However, this practice should not be undertaken prior to many years of training to reach one's "natural potential". Nonetheless, both protein supplementation and creatine monohydrate supplementation in youth should be monitored by a physician who determines kidney and liver function. β-alanine, sodium bicarbonate, caffeine, sports drinks, oral rehydration solutions, and concentrated carbohydrate solutions can be used successfully to improve performance. Particular caution should be taken with caffeine, although ergogenic, it can contribute to dehydration.

ETHICAL CONSIDERATIONS FOR THE USE OF DIETARY SUPPLEMENTS IN YOUTH

Clearly, the research on the safety of dietary supplements in youth is behind the research in adults. Without safety data to go on, we have to use logic and make sure the youth are not harmed by taking Dietary Supplements. We may ask what is the harm if the youth do not take the Dietary Supplement. The answer is in some cases it is a nutritional deficiency. Parnell, Wiens, and Erdman et al. (2016) found that youth athletes were deficient in Vitamin D and potassium. Clearly, this would suggest that youth should supplement vitamin D (so as not to develop a deficiency). Potassium supplementation from a cardiac standpoint should probably take the form of eating more fruit, particularly bananas. Let us turn to protein supplementation. The protein needs of adult resistance trained athletes is on the order of ~1.6 g/kg bodyweight/day (Lemon et al. 1992). The protein needs, i.e., Recommended Daily Allowance (RDA) for adolescents is similar to that of adults. It follows then, logically, that if adult resistance trained athletes need ~1.6 g/kg bodyweight/day then so would adolescent resistance trained athletes. We have no reason to believe that a young kidney is less tolerant of protein than an adult kidney. However, if a youth athlete takes in this quantity of protein, they should likely have their kidney function checked by a physician, and this simply involves drawing a blood sample (for creatinine and blood urea nitrogen). That being said, it is hard to take in that quantity of protein(1.6 g/kg/day) without supplementation. Thus, I believe there is a case for protein supplements in youth athletes.

Creatine monohydrate is highly ergogenic in adults and is presently being used in clinical trials of youth muscle disease (Banerjee et al. 2010; Kley et al. 2013). Creatine besides being effective in improving muscle mass, strength, and muscular endurance has been shown to be safe in adults. Again, this Nutritional Dietary Supplement is legal in international competition (i.e., not banned by the World Antidoping Agency (WADA). The argument being that nutritional knowledge is power and good nutrition is not cheating. Clearly, there is much athletic potential to be realized before legal nutritional ergogenic aids should be utilized. Therefore, I believe adolescent athletes could use creatine monohydrate ethically but should have liver and kidney function routinely assessed by a physician.

NUTRITIONAL SUPPLEMENTS AND THE HIGH-PERFORMANCE ADULT (>18 YEARS OF AGE) WRESTLER

For a thorough discussion of dietary supplements and the high-performance athlete, see the IOC Position stand lead authored by Ron Maughan, PhD (Maughan et al. 2018). This article is expansive and complete on the topic of dietary supplements and adult athletes. The review includes the way scientists evaluate research studies to determine their validity (accuracy) and reliability (consistency). Supplements likely to be effective in the adult amateur wrestler are High Carbohydrate Supplements, Protein, Creatine Monohydrate, β-Alanine, Sodium Bicarbonate, Caffeine, Sports Drinks, and Oral Rehydration Solutions.

SUPPLEMENTS THAT ARE LIKELY EFFECTIVE IN AMATEUR WRESTLING AND NOT BANNED BY WADA

PROTEIN SUPPLEMENTS

To obtain the required amount of protein without the extra fat calories athletes may have to take in Protein Supplements. There are numerous kinds of protein supplements on the market, with Whey and Casein being the most popular. Whey protein in addition to being a rich source of essential amino acids has antioxidant properties which may help stave off muscle fatigue (Hu and Zemel 2003). Casein is a milk protein that breaks down slower than Whey, providing a less dramatic increase but a sustained increase in muscle protein synthesis (Tipton et al. 2004).

CONCENTRATED CARBOHYDRATE SUPPLEMENTS

Although the author is aware of few if any concentrated carbohydrate supplements on the market, this would appear to be a beneficial supplement for those engaged in

2–3 hour practices per day. The quantity of carbohydrate derived from whole foods is almost impossible to eat when trying to support a 4,000–5,000 kcal/day diet which may be required for optimal performance when practicing 2–3 h/day. My point is, simple sugars are ok to ingest if you are going to burn them in practice. To eat enough calories for these prolonged practices it is imperative that condensed products with simple sugars are ingested to supply enough calories to train optimally. Foods and beverages such as sugary cereals, low-fat chocolate milk, and grape juice would appear to be good choices.

CREATINE MONOHYDRATE

Creatine is a substance derived from amino acids and is used in the reaction Creatine + ATP $\diamondsuit$ PCr + ADP. Paul Greenhaff, Roger Harris, Eric Hultman, and their co-authors (Greenhaff et al. 1993; Birch et al. 1994; Casey et al. 1996) were the first ones to research creatine and found that it elevates Phosphocreatine (PCr) in skeletal muscle and improves intermittent high-intensity exercise performance (Greenhaff et al. 1993; Birch et al. 1994; Casey et al. 1996). The typical protocol for supplementing creatine is 20 g/day for 5 days. That is 4×5 g/day for 5 days. This loading protocol's effects last for 1 month. The mechanism of action is elevated PCr stores and possibly an enhanced rate of PCr resynthesis between exercise bouts (Greenhaff et al. 1994).

β-ALANINE

High-intensity exercise of intermittent or relatively short duration has been shown to be augmented by β-Alanine supplementation. β-Alanine acts to increase the muscle buffering substance called carnosine in skeletal muscle. Carnosine is a powerful buffer. The protocol for β-Alanine ingestion is 4–6 g per day for 4 weeks. The only known side effect of supplementation with β-Alanine is a tingling in the face and neck regions (Trexler et al. 2015).

SODIUM BICARBONATE

Also known as $NaHCO_3$, Sodium Bicarbonate is an extracellular buffer. In many instances Sodium Bicarbonate given at 0.3 g/kg bodyweight or less (Costill et al. 1984) has been shown to improve high-intensity intermittent exercise performance. The proposed mechanism for this improvement in high-intensity exercise performance is an improved efflux of H^+ from skeletal muscle, thus lessening the effect of these hydrogen ions on fatigue mechanisms within the muscle. One potential side effect of Sodium Bicarbonate ingestion is diarrhea. It must be noted that sodium bicarbonate is not always performance enhancing and much of this depends on the exercise paradigm or protocol.

CAFFEINE

Coffee and other drinks contain caffeine and the effects of caffeine at high doses (700–900 mg; 5–7 cups of coffee) on improvements in exercise performance have been established and are not banned by WADA (Maughan et al. 2018). However, there are side effects associated with such high dosages such as diarrhea and nausea. Lower doses of caffeine ~200 mg have also been shown to be ergogenic but without the associated side effects. The mechanism of action with low-dose caffeine appears to reside in the central nervous system (Spriet et al. 2014).

SPORTS DRINKS

Carbohydrate–electrolyte drinks called sports drinks are a great boon to training. First, they aid in rehydration because the carbohydrates and sodium in the drink aid in intestinal absorption and retention of fluids in the body after ingestion (Evans, Shirreffs, and Maughan 2009, 2011). Second, sports drinks also augment exercise performance during events lasting greater than 1 hour such as a wrestling practice and therefore will improve the gains in performance seen by one and many training sessions.

ORAL REHYDRATION SOLUTIONS

Oral Rehydration Solutions are important when an individual is dehydrated such as after practice. These solutions in addition to containing about half the carbohydrate (adequate to increase intestinal absorption) as Sports Drinks contain about 3–5 times as much sodium (~43–90 mmol/L sodium) as Sports Drinks. This clearly is set up to maximally stimulate intestinal absorption and augment fluid retention within the vascular system and total body water pool. Additionally, these solutions are hypotonic so they tend to empty from the stomach faster than Sports Drinks. Examples of such drinks are Pedialyte and Dioralyte (Table 24.1).

TABLE 24.1

Selected Nutritional Ergogenic Aids and Effects

Supplement	Purported Function
Protein supplements	Improved muscle protein synthesis after training sessions relative to carbohydrate alone or fasting
Concentrated carbohydrate solutions	Improved muscle glycogen resynthesis after training sessions compared with protein supplements or fasting or sports drinks (Burke et al. 1994; Kersick et al. 2008)
Sports drinks	Assists in rehydration and sustains carbohydrate oxidation during exercise.
Oral rehydration solutions	Optimize rehydration during and after exercise (Evans, Shirreffs, and Maughan 2009, 2011)
Creatine monohydrate	Enhances intermittent high-intensity exercise performance by increasing PCr stores (Greenhaff et al. 1993; Birch et al. 1994; Casey et al. 1996)
β-Alanine	Enhances intermittent high-intensity exercise performance by increasing muscle carnosine levels and therefore muscle buffering capacity (Trexler et al. 2015)
Sodium bicarbonate	Enhances intermittent high-intensity exercise performance by improving extracellular buffering capacity (Costill et al. 1984)
Caffeine	Central nervous system stimulant can improve maximal force generating capacity by improving "psychological arousal" (Maughan et al. 2018; Spriet 2014)

KEY POINTS

1. Nutritional ergogenic aids are effective and legal (within federal and state laws and within the rules of sport) means to improve exercise performance.
2. Protein supplements, creatine, and caffeine can be taken by youth but should be done under the supervision of a physician.
3. Other effective and safe supplements are Concentrated Carbohydrate Solutions, Sports Drinks, Oral rehydration solutions, β-alanine, and sodium bicarbonate.
4. Clearly, with 2–4 hours of practice in a day Concentrated Carbohydrate Solutions (such as sugary cereal and milk, grape juice, low-fat chocolate milk) are warranted due to the high carbohydrate turnover of such long practice sessions.

25 Relative Energy Deficiency in Sport (RED-S)

Relative Energy Deficiency in Sport (RED-S) is a phenomenon that is caused by two factors: reduced energy intake and increased energy output. It occurs in both men and women. It results in reduced exercise performance capabilities, reduced protein synthesis, and altered hormone levels which could lead to, for example, amenorrhea in women. Under the current high-school guidelines of being allowed to lose 1.5% of bodyweight per week during the season it is quite possible that RED-S could happen in high-school and collegiate athletes.

RELATIVE ENERGY DEFICIENCY IN SPORT

A recent phenomenon has been discovered, which increases our understanding of the effects of reduced energy availability in addition to understanding of the effect of reduced carbohydrate availability on exercise performance. It is called Relative Energy Deficiency in Sport RED-S. RED-S affects both men and women (Mountjoy et al. 2018a,b). It extends our knowledge of the effects of reduced energy availability not only on performance but also on negatively altered hormone levels and protein synthesis rates. There are two factors that lead to RED-S or its precursor Low Energy Availability: Decreased energy intake and/or increased exercise load (Table 25.1).

In a sport such as wrestling which has weight classes and wrestlers are always trying to reach an optimal body composition for performance, reduced energy intake is a major factor. Additionally, with 1.5–3.0 hour practices ~5 days/week, a high exercise load is another factor but training load could stay constant if energy intake was adequate. However, with athletes allowed to lose 1.5% of bodyweight per week or about 1.5–3.0 lbs/week (2.31 lbs/week for the 154 lbs reference man) to reach a weight class, energy intake is likely inadequate (energy intake is ~1,155 calories

---

TABLE 25.1

Causes of RED-S

Reduced energy intake

Increased energy expenditure

[a]A combination of reduced energy intake and increased energy expenditure

[a] Most likely scenario

---

below weight maintenance/day) to maintain carbohydrate balance, protein balance, and exercise performance at optimal levels for 1.5–3 hours ~5 days/week with resting metabolism being about ~1,706 kcal/day (Harris–Benedict Formula 1918), thermic effect of feeding being ~171 kcal/day, and exercise energy expenditure being about ~1,600 kcal/day (~800 kcal/day × 2 hours) for a grand total energy expenditure of 3,477 kcal/day needed to maintain bodyweight. To lose 2.31 lbs per week or 1.5% of bodyweight would be a reduction of ~1,155 kcal/day, leaving the athlete at an energy intake of 2322 kcal/day. At 60% CHO (348 g CHO; 5.0 g/kg CHO), 20% PRO (116g; 1.66 g/kg PRO), and 20% FAT (52 g of FAT; 5.8 g/kg FAT). Clearly, this is an inadequate amount of carbohydrate (5.0 g/kg) to fuel wrestling performances which should be about 8.0–10 g/kg bodyweight per day. Indeed, Costill et al. (1988) found that swimmers who did not consume ~8 g/kg CHO/day were unable to maintain training volume and intensity during a period of intensified training. This is supported by data in runners from the same laboratory in which 3.9 g/kg/day of carbohydrate was insufficient to maintain muscle glycogen stores in trained runners during intensified training (Kirwan et al. 1988). This would likely be the case because the wrestlers would be in negative energy and carbohydrate balance which would result in impaired high-intensity exercise performance. This is because 3.9 g/kg CHO would be inadequate to replace muscle and liver glycogen stores. Additionally, the effects of prolonged periods of time in a reduced energy (calorie) state could lead to RED-S. This is because the athlete is below their body fat set point. How long an athlete can be below their body fat set point or how much below the body fat set point an athlete can be before developing RED-S is unknown. A much more prudent strategy for losing weight would be dieting and long slow-distance exercise to burn fat *before* the season when fueling with carbohydrate and rebuilding muscle degraded during practice with protein is less crucial. Even if an athlete changes the macronutrient composition of their diet to more favorable one for athletic performance, say 60% CHO, 20% Protein, and 20% Fat from their normal diet (Normal American diet 50% CHO, 15% Protein, and 35% Fat), this will not adequately allow for recovery between exercise bouts if in *negative energy* and *carbohydrate balance*. Thus, to reiterate it is best for the wrestler to lose the weight before the season and maintain weight and exercise performance by eating a high-carbohydrate diet during the season. The current guidelines of losing 1.5% of bodyweight per week during the season would result in inadequate carbohydrate nutrition during the season to maintain and optimize wrestling anaerobic and aerobic performance. However, the magnitude of this problem depends on practice length. Losing 1.5% of bodyweight per week may not be that drastic if practices are not too extreme in length. Clearly, excessive training has problems in and of itself. It is possible and potentially probable that you can "outrun your diet". In the studies of Costill et al. (1988) in swimmers and Kirwan et al. (1988) in runners, a portion of the athletes could not maintain training intensity with a doubling of training volume. In the study of Costill et al. (1988) the swimmers who could tolerate the increase in volume ingested 8.2 gCHO/kg/day and the swimmers who could not tolerate the increase in volume ingested 5.3 gCHO/kg/day. In the study of Kirwan et al. (1988) the subjects ingested either 8.0 gCHO/kg/day or 3.9 gCHO/kg/day during intensified running training. Even on the 8.0 g/kg/day muscle glycogen stores were suboptimal. The studies of Costill et al. (1988) and

TABLE 25.2
Symptoms of RED-S

Women	Men
	Reduced Exercise Performance
Altered female reproductive hormones (IOC Position Stand on RED-S 2018)	Altered male reproductive and growth hormones/factors (Roemmich and Sinning 1987a,b)
Potentially the female athlete triad resulting in reduced energy intake, amenorrhea, reduced bone density, as well as reduced muscle protein synthesis (IOC Position Stand on RED-S 2018)	Unknown to a large extent but clearly would result in reduced muscle protein synthesis. Could result in reduced long bone growth and reduced bone density

Kirwan et al. (1988) were practical from the standpoint of how much swimmers and runners train. The take-home message is that a very high carbohydrate diet needs to be eaten with such training or there needs to be reduction in training volume. Eating 8 g CHO/kg bodyweight/day is no easy task. For the 154 lb wrestler (70 kg) this is 560 g of carbohydrate per day. Thus, it is almost a must that simple carbohydrate has to be taken in to fill the requirements from a food volume standpoint. Another take-home message is one of excessive training. If one trains less they can take in less carbohydrate for optimal performance. What we don't know in wrestlers is if their training loads are excessive. Excessive training leads to a reduction in free testosterone, total testosterone, and dehydroepiandrosterone sulphate (DHEA-S) (Flynn et al. 1997). What is not clear from Flynn et al.'s data is the role of diet in this study. Thus, from the studies of Costill et al. (1988), Kirwan et al. (1988), and Flynn, Pizza, and Brolinson (1997) it is unclear whether they are training too much and/or eating too little presumably carbohydrate. The mechanism for the reduction in male hormones needs to be elucidated; is it excessive training, inadequate nutrition, or both. Also, Fitts, Costill, and Gardetto (1989) reported a reduction in type II (fast twitch glycolytic) fiber diameter during excessive training. The question arises: Is inadequate nutrition and/or a reduction in male hormones that cause this reduction in type II fiber diameter (Table 25.2).

KEY POINTS

1. RED-S is a problem for both male and female athletes and likely for wrestlers. However, the extent of the problem in wrestling is unknown.
2. The current guideline of allowing a weight loss of 1.5% per week in high-school and collegiate wrestling may be adding to the problem of RED-S due to inadequate carbohydrate intake during periods of weight loss and heavy training (Costill et al. 1988; Kirwan et al. 1988).
3. RED-S manifests itself in inadequate energy intake, changes in hormones in both men and women, amenorrhea in women, and potential changes in muscle protein synthesis and bone density.

4. A prudent recommendation for weight loss is to lose fat at a rate of 1–2 lbs/week before the season and maintain weight with a 60% carbohydrate, 20% protein, and 20% fat diet during the season. This will allow for optimal performances on the mat during the season, which likely would not be afforded if losing 1.5% bodyweight per week during the season.

26 Special Considerations for the Female Wrestler

Female wrestlers are a unique breed, indeed. Additionally, they are prone to the Female Athlete Triad which is reduced energy availability (EA), amenorrhea, and reduced bone mineral density. A major factor in the Female Athlete Triad is Relative Energy Deficiency in Sport (RED-S; Mountjoy et al. 2018a,b). This is a relative imbalance between energy output and energy intake (EI) or excessive exercise coupled with reduced EI. A question arises with regard to female wrestlers: should they lift weights? The answer is a resounding yes. High correlations have been found in women between whole body fat-free mass and time to fatigue at 100% of VO_2max an intensity and duration that is similar to a wrestling match. That is the more muscle they had, the more fatigue resistant they were.

The female wrestler is a unique athlete. As will be discussed energy balance and weight maintenance are extremely important. Women and adolescent girl athletes are prone to the female athlete triad (Mountjoy et al. 2018a,b; IOC Position Stand 2018). This triad consists of reduced EA (International Olympic Committee [IOC] position stand), ammenhorea, and reduced bone mineral density. The major contributing factor to the female athlete triad is RED-S. This could be caused by excessive energy expenditure and/or inadequate EI (IOC position stand). The most important line of attack against RED-S and the Female Athlete Triad is prevention. This should encompass collecting continuous food log data and keeping a continuous exercise diary as well as determining fat-free mass (and possibly body weight) on a routine basis. EA is calculated as EI minus daily energy costs of exercise relative to fat-free mass. According to the IOC working group, a value for EA of 45 kcal/kg ffm/day equates to energy balance in healthy adults. So too little EI and/or much little training can put the person in RED-S and can lead to the Female Athlete Triad. RED-S may likely be defined by relative carbohydrate deficiency in athletes as carbohydrate is the main substrate for intense exercise. Early research from Costill's Group at Ball State University in male swimmers suggests that the swimmers who could not keep up with 10 days of intensified training did not eat sufficient carbohydrate. Those that tolerated the swimming stress took in 8 g/kg bodyweight/day while those that did not tolerate increased swim volume took in 5 g/kg bodyweight/day (Costill et al. 1988). Similar results were found in male runners from the same laboratory (Kirwan et al. 1988). These results need to be replicated in male and female wrestlers.

SHOULD WOMEN LIFT WEIGHTS FOR WRESTLING?

The answer to this is a resounding yes. Lambert et al. (2013) examined the relationship between fat-free mass and time to fatigue at 100% of VO_2 max (somewhat similar duration to a wrestling match as far as energy systems are concerned) and found that 48% of the variability in time to fatigue could be attributed to whole body fat-free mass in these recreationally trained men and women. Since muscle mass is a surrogate for muscle strength, high muscle strength is likely the determinant of longer duration on this time to fatigue test. Therefore, yes strength is important to wrestling muscular endurance and women should lift weights for this reason in addition to the effects on muscle strength itself. Using logic, if resistance training is safe for children, which it is, it would also be safe for women who also have relatively low testosterone compared to their male counterparts.

KEY POINTS

1. Female athletes should train in much the same way as male athletes.
2. Resistance training should be a staple of a female wrestler's training regimen as maximal force development would appear to be a strong component of wrestling success.
3. Female and Male athletes are prone to RED-S.
4. Female athletes with RED-S are prone to amenorrhea and bone loss. Therefore, much effort should be put forth to make sure this phenomenon does not occur in female athletes.
5. The syndrome that occurs in male athletes is much less known but theoretically could also lead to bone loss.
6. RED-S may likely be due to carbohydrate energy insufficiency, and therefore carbohydrate should be ingested to match the energy output of training at 8–10 g carbohydrate/kg bodyweight (Table 26.1).

TABLE 26.1

Female-Related Problems and Solutions to Optimize Competitive Wrestling

Problems	Solutions
RED-S	Stay in energy balance during the competitive season (bodyweight and food diaries)
Low muscle strength	Training with weights similar to men will not only increase strength but will likely will increase fatigue resistance (Lambert et al. 2013) and may increase VO_2peak (Lambert 2020).

---

27 Weight Control and Physical Fitness in the Years after a Wrestler's Competitive Career

The major change that occurs after the wrestler's competitive career is a reduction in energy output as practices have ceased. This results in weight gain if the former athlete does not reduce energy intake or partake in regular physical activity. Clearly, some weight gain is probable, and in many former wrestlers, a considerable weight gain is probable. Taking up a regular physical activity in the years after the competitive career and eating prudently are remedies to such weight gain. Other interventions could be behavioral or psychological as the attachment of food is probable as a result of times of extreme deprivation during their wrestling career.

Clearly energy output (exercise) goes down immediately after the competitive career of the wrestler. The decrease in the energy (kcals) expended is great and can be on the order of ~1,320 kcals for each day of lack of training. This is the equivalent of a gain of 2.65 lbs (1.2 kg) per week for an average wrestler who becomes sedentary after his competitive career. Clearly, this high rate of weight gain will not go indefinitely but is certainly an important consideration. If energy intake stays the same as when in the competitive career this compounds the problem greatly. Assuming most individuals need 2,000 kcal per day in a sedentary existence and covering energy expenditure during the competitive career, this would be an energy need of ~3,320 kcals per day to stay in energy balance for competition. Thus, eating as if you were competing when in post-competitive period will increase body fat levels (as a result of a positive energy balance). What then must an athlete in his post-competitive years do to maintain a healthy weight and not become overweight. (1) Maintain a regular exercise program including calorie burning activities such as walking, cycling, or running. This is supported by research suggesting that high cardiorespiratory fitness is a negative predictor of mortality (Ross et al. 2016). (2) Reduce energy intake (kcals) by keeping calories relatively low (i.e., 2,000 kcal/day for a sedentary person). A pound of fat is 3,500 kcal in excess of needs. This would mean avoiding fatty foods (9 kcal/gram), and more than two alcoholic drinks per day (7 kcal/g of alcohol). Clearly, if on an exercise program, you could eat more than 2,000 kcals/day if you burn at least 500 kcals/day in regular physical exercise. Additionally, research has shown that aerobic exercise of relatively long duration (60 min/day) will reduce the propensity for type II diabetes presumably by reducing the stores of muscle glycogen. The study participants in this study were on a 50%

TABLE 27.1

Problems and Solutions to Problems That Occur in the Post-Competitive Decades

Problems	Solutions
Weight gain	Exercise 3–6 days/week and eat a low-fat diet to maintain energy balance
Increase in cardiovascular risk factors	Exercise 3–6 days/week and eat a low-fat diet to maintain energy balance

CHO diet of about 2,000 kcal/day (Arciero et al. 1999). The exercise in this study was of moderate intensity, i.e., the subjects could likely talk during exercise. One alternative to this paradigm would be to become a weekend warrior. That is to get involved in marathon running, tour cycling, wrestling refereeing, indoor or outdoor soccer, and hiking. In this scenario, the kcals for intake could be significantly more without gaining weight, i.e., maintenance of energy balance. The exercise should be done year round. Lifelong exercise is an excellent option for maintaining Physical Fitness, as assessed my maximal oxygen consumption and preventing cardiovascular disease. Data on large populations of various fitness levels suggest duration on a treadmill during a treadmill stress test is predictive of all cause mortality (if you are going to die from all causes.). Thus, being physically fit is more important than having a low fat percentage with regard to cardiovascular disease (Ross et al. 2019). Recently, the importance of muscular endurance to prevent cardiovascular disease has come to light. These investigators found that those individuals who could perform 40 pushups in 60 seconds were almost devoid of cardiovascular disease (Yang et al. 2019). Therefore, there also appears to be a role for resistance exercise (weight training) in the prevention of cardiovascular disease. In this case, it is likely that you might be "fit and fat" as resistance exercise typically does not burn many calories (Table 27.1).

KEY POINTS: POST-COMPETITIVE CAREER CONSIDERATIONS

1. Due to the reduction in energy output a wrestler is likely to gain a moderate amount of weight after his competitive career.
2. To combat this weight gain, one should exercise regularly (3–6 times per week) and attempt to go on a weight maintenance energy (calorie) intake.
3. It is quite possible for one to remain fit and be fat and as a result have low potential for developing cardiovascular disease. Regular physical exercise is anti-inflammatory and this has a positive effect on cardiovascular health.
4. Additionally, recent data suggests that strength training that leads to excellent muscular endurance (40 pushups in a row) leads to reduced risk of cardiovascular disease.

References

ACSM. ACSM guidelines for fluid delivery. In: *ACSM Guidelines for Exercise Testing and Prescription*, 9th Edition, 456 p. Senior Ed: Pescatello LS. Philadelphia, PA: Wolters Kluwer/Lippincott Williams and Wilkins, 2014.

Andersen LL, Tufekovic G, Zebis MK, Crameri RM, Verlaan G, Kjaer M, Suetta C, Magnusson P, Aagaard P. The effect of resistance training combined with timed ingestion of protein on muscle fiber size and strength. *Metabolism* 54:151–156, 2005.

Aragon A, Schoenfeld BJ, Wildman R, Kleiner S, VanDusseldorp T, Taylor L, Earnest CP, Arciero PJ, Wilborn C, Kalman DS, Stout JR. International Society of Sports Nutrition Position Stand: diets and body composition. *J. Int. Soc. Sports Nutr.* 14:16, 2017.

Arciero PJ, Vukovich MD, Holloszy JO, Racette SB, Kohrt WM. Comparison of short-term diet and exercise on insulin action in individuals with abnormal glucose tolerance. *J. Appl. Physiol.* 86:1930–1935, 1999.

Armstrong LE, Costill DL, Fink WJ. Influence of diuretic-induced dehydration on competitive running performance. *Med. Sci. Sports Exerc.* 17:456–461, 1985.

Baker LB, De Chavez PJD, Ungaro CT, Sopena BC, Nuccia RP, Reimel AJ, Barnes KA. Exercise intensity effects on total sweat electrolyte losses and regional vs. whole-body sweat $[Na^+]$, $[Cl^-]$, and $[K^+]$. *Eur. J. Appl. Physiol.* 119:361–375, 2019.

Ball D, Greenhaff PL, Maughan RJ. The acute reversal of a diet induced metabolic acidosis does not restore endurance capacity during high intensity exercise in man. *Eur. J. Appl. Physiol.* 73(1–2):105–112, 1996.

Behm DG, Sale DG. Intended rather than actual movement velocity determines velocity-specific training response. *J. Appl. Physiol.* 74:359–368, 1993.

Borg G. Psychophysical bases of perceived exertion. *Med. Sci. Sports Exerc.* 14:377–381, 1982.

Brooks GA, Fahey TD, Baldwin KM. *Exercise Physiology: Human Bioenergetics and Its Applications*, 4th Edition. Boston, MA: McGraw-Hill, 2005.

Banerjee B, Sharma U, Balasubramanian K, Kalaivani M, Kalra V, Jagannathan NR. Effect of creatine monohydrate in improving cellular energetics and muscle strength in ambulatory Duchenne muscular dystrophy patients: a randomized, placebo-controlled 31P MRS study. *Magn. Reson. Imaging* 28(5):698–707, 2010. doi: 10.1016/j.mri.2010.03.008. Epub 2010 April 15.

Below PR, Mora-Rodriguez R, Gonzalez-Alonso J, Coyle EF. Fluid and carbohydrate ingestion independently improve performance during 1H of intense exercise. *Med. Sci. Sports Exerc.* 27:200–210, 1995.

Bergstrom J, Hermansen L, Hultman E, Saltin B. Diet, muscle glycogen and physical performance. *Acta Phys. Scand.* 71:140–150, 1967.

Bergstrom J, Hultman E. A study of the glycogen metabolism during exercise in man. *Scand. J.Clin. Lab. Invest.* 19:218–228, 1967.

Bigard AX, Sanchez H, Claveyolas G, Martin S, Thimonier B, Arnaud MT. Effects of dehydration and rehydration on EMG changes during fatiguing contractions. *Med. Sci. Sports Exerc.* 33:1694–1700, 2001.

Birch R Noble D, Greenhaff PL. The influence of daily creatine supplementation on performance during repeated bouts of maximal isokinetic cycling in man. *Eur. J. App. Physiol.* 69:268–276, 1994.

Born KA, Dooley EE, Cheshire PA, McGill CC, Cosgrove JM, Ivy JL, Bartholomew JB. Chocolate milk versus carbohydrate supplements in adolescent athletes: a field based study. *J. Int. Soc. Sport Nutr.* 16:6, 2019. doi: 10.1186/s12976-019-0272-0.

Bowtell JC, Leese GP, Smith K, Watt PM, Nevill AM, Rooyakers O, Wagenmackers ATM, Rennie MJ. Effect of oral glucose on leucine turnover in humans at rest and during exercise at two levels of dietary protein. *J. Physiol.* 525(1):271–281, 2000.

Burke LM, Collier GR, Hargreaves M. Muscle glycogen storage after prolonged exercise: effect of the glycemic index of carbohydrate feedings. *J. Appl. Physiol.* 75:1019–1023, 1993.

Burke LM, Ross ML, Garvican-Lewis LA, Welvaert M, Heikura JA, Forbes SG, Mirtschin JG, Catol E, Strobel N, Sharma AP, Hawley JA. Low carbohydrate, high fat diet impairs exercise economy and negates the performance benefit from intensified training in elite race walkers. *J. Physiol.* 595:2785–2807, 2017.

Caldwell JE, Ahonen E, Nousiamen U. Differential effects of sauna-, diuretic, and exercise induced hypohydration. *J. Appl. Physiol.* 57:1018–1023, 1984.

Casey A, Constantin-Teodosiu D, Howell S, Hultman E, Greenhaff PL. Creatine ingestion favorably affects performance and muscle metabolism during maximal exercise. *Am. J. Physiol.* 271(1 pt 1):E31–E37, 1996.

Caterisano A, Camaione DN, Murphy RT, Gomino VJ. The effect of different training on isokinetic muscular endurance during acute thermally induced hypohydration. *Am. J. Sports Med.* 16:269–273, 1988.

Cheuvront SN, Carter R, Haymes EM, Sawka MK. No effect of moderate hypohydration or hyperthermia on anaerobic exercise performance. *Med. Sci. Sports Exerc.* 38:1093–1097, 2006.

Cleary MA, Hetzler RK, Wasson D, Wages JJ, Stickley C, Kimura IF. Hydration behaviors before and after an educational and prescribed hydration intervention in adolescent athletes. *J. Athl. Train.* 47:273–281, 2012.

Coggan AR, Coyle EF. Reversal of the fatigue during prolonged exercise by carbohydrate infusion or ingestion. *J. Appl. Physiol.* 63:2388–2395, 1987.

Colbert BJ, Ankney JJ, Lee KT. *Anatomy, Physiology, & Disease: An Interactive Journey for Health Professionals*, 3rd Edition. New York, NY: Pearson, 2020.

Constantin-Teodosiu D, Cederblad G, Bergstrom M, Greenhaff PL. Maximal-intensity exercise does not fully restore muscle pyruvate dehydrogenase complex activation after 3 days of high-fat dietary intake. *Clin. Nutr.* 38:948–953, 2019.

Cooper KH. A means of assessing maximal oxygen uptake. *JAMA.* 203:201–204, 1968.

Costill DL. Sweating: its composition and effect on body fluids. *Ann. NY Acad. Sci.* 301:160–174, 1977.

Costill DL, Bennett A, Branam G, Eddy D. Glucose ingestion at rest and during prolonged exercise. *J. Appl. Physiol.* 34:764–769, 1973.

Costill DL, Flynn MG, Kirwan JP, Houmard JA, Mitchell JB, Thomas R, Park SH. Effects of repeated days of intensified training on muscle glycogen and swimming performance. *Med. Sci. Sports Exerc.* 20:249–254, 1988.

Costill DL, Thomas R, Robergs RA, Pascoe D, Lambert C, Barr S, Fink WJ. Adaptations to swimming training: influence of training volume. *Med. Sci. Sports Exerc.* 23:371–377, 1991.

Costill DL, Saltin B. Factors limiting gastric emptying during rest and exercise. *J. Appl. Physiol.* 37:679–683, 1974.

Costill DL, Verstappen F, Kuipers H, Janssen E, Fink W. Acid-base balance during repeated bouts of exercise: influence of HCO_3^-. *Int. J. Sports Med.* 5:228–231, 1984.

DeFronzo RA, Ferrannini E, Sato Y, Felig P, Wahren J. Synergistic interaction between exercise and insulin on peripheral glucose uptake. *J. Clin. Invest.* 68:1468–1474, 1981.

Delorme TL, Watkins AL. Technics of progressive resistance exercise. *Arch. Phys. Med. Rehab.* 29:263–273, 1948.

Donnely J, Hillman C, Castelli P, et al. ACSM Position Stand on physical activity, cognitive function, and academic achievement in children. *Med. Sci. Sports Exerc.* 48:1223–1224, 2016.

Dotan R, Bar-Or O. Load optimization for the Wingate anaerobic test. *Eur. J. Appl. Physiol.* 51:409–417, 1983.

Dubowitz VMHB, Neville, HE. *Muscle Biopsy: A Modern Approach.* Vol. 2 in the series "Major Problems in Neurology". Philadelphia, PA: W.B. Saunders Company Ltd., 1973.

Enoka RM. *Neuromechanics of Human Movement.* Champaign, IL: Human Kinetics, 2008.

Evans GH, Shirreffs SM, Maughan RJ. Post-exercise rehydration in man the effects of carbohydrate content and osmolality of the drink ingested ad libitum. *Appl. Physiol. Nutr. Metab.* 34:783–785, 2009.

Evans GH, Shirreffs SM, Maughan RJ. The effect of repeated ingestion of high and low glucose-electrolyte solutions on gastric emptying and blood $2H_2O$ concentrations after an overnight fast. *Br. Nutr.* 106:1732–1739, 2011.

Fitts RH, Costill DL, Gardetto PR. Effect of swim exercise training on human muscle fiber function. *J. Appl. Physiol.* 66:465–475, 1989.

Fleming J, Sharman MJ, Avery NG, Love AM, Gomez AL, Scheett TP, Kraemer WJ, Volek JS. Endurance capacity and high intensity exercise performance responses to a high fat diet. *Int. J. Sport Nutr. Exerc. Metab.* 13:466–478, 2003.

Flynn MG, Michaud TJ, Rodriguez-Zayas J, Lambert CP, Boone JB, Mosleski RW. Effect of 4-and 8-h pre-exercise feedings on substrate use and performance. *J. Appl. Physiol.* 67:2066–2071, 1989.

Flynn MG, Pizza FX, Brolinson PG. Hormonal responses to excessive training: influence of cross training. *Int. J. Sports Med.* 18:191–196, 1997.

Foster C, Costill DL, Fink WJ. Effects of pre-exercise feedings on endurance performance. *Med. Sci. Sports* 11:1–5, 1979.

Foster-Powell K, Holt SHA, Brand-Miller JC. International table of glycemic index and glycemic load values: 2002. *Am. J. Clin. Nutr.* 76:5–56, 2002.

Friedlander AL, Braun B, Pollack M, Macdonald JB, Fulco CS, Muza SR, Rock PB, Henderson GC, Horning MA, Brooks GA, Hoffman AR, Cymerman A. Three weeks of caloric restriction alters protein metabolism in normal weight young men. *Am. J. Physiol. Endocrinol. Metab.* 289:E446–E455, 2005.

Fryburg DA, Barrett EJ, Louard RJ, Gelfand RA. Fffect of starvation on human protein metabolism and the response to insulin. *Am. J. Physiol.* 259:E477–E482, 1990.

Gibala MG, MacDougall JD, Sale DG. The effects of tapering on strength performance in trained athletes. *Int. J. Sports Med.* 15:492–497, 1994.

Gibbs AE, Pickemann J, Sekiya JK. Weight management in amateur wrestling. *Sports Health* 1:227–230, 2009.

Gleeson M, Greenhaff PL, Maughan RJ. Influence of a 24 hour fast on high-intensity cycle exercise performance in man. *Eur. J. Appl. Physiol.* 57:653–659, 1988.

Godek SF, Bartolozzi AR, Burkholder R, Sugarman E, Peduzzi C. Sweat rates and fluid turnover in professional football players: a comparison of National Football League linemen and backs. *J. Athl. Train.* 43:184–189, 2008.

Gollnick PD, Armstrong RB, Sembrowich WL, Shepherd RE, Saltin, B. Glycogen depletion patterns in human skeletal muscle after heavy exercise. *J. Appl. Physiol.* 34:615–618, 1973.

Green HJ. Metabolic determinants of activity induced muscular fatigue. In: *Exercise Metabolism*, pp. 211–256. Ed: Hargreaves M, Champaign: Human Kinetics, 2005.

Greenhaff PL, Bodin K, Soderlund K, Hultman E. Effect of oral creatine supplementation on skeletal muscle phosphocreatine resynthesis. *Am. J. Physiol.* 266:E725–E730, 1994.

Greenhaff PL, Casey A, Short AA, Harris R, Soderlund K, Hultman E. Influence of oral creatine supplementation on muscle torque during repeated bouts of maximal voluntary exercise in man. *Clin. Sci.* 84:565–571, 1993.

Greenhaff PL, Gleeson M, Maughan RJ. Diet induced metabolic acidosis and the performance of high intensity exercise in man. *Eur. J. Appl. Physiol.* 57:583–590, 1988a.

Greenhaff PL, Gleeson M, Maughan RJ. The effects of diet on muscle pH and metabolism during high intensity exercise. *Eur. J. Appl. Physiol.* 57:531–539, 1988b.

Gutierrez A, Mesa JL, Ruiz JR, Chirosa CJ, Castillo MJ. Sauna-induced rapid weight loss decreases explosive power in women but not in men. *Int. J. Sports Med.* 24:518–522, 2003.

Guyton AC, Hall JE. *Textbook of Medical Physiology*, 11th Edition. Philadelphia, PA: Elsevier Saunders, 2006.

Ha E, Zemel MB. Functional properties whey, whey constituents, and essential amino acids: mechanisms underlying health and disease for active people (review). *J. Nutr. Biochem.* 14:251–258, 2003.

Halson S, Jones D. Detecting and avoiding overtraining. In: *High-Performance Cycling*, pp. 13–16. Ed: Jeukendrup AE. Champaign, IL: Human Kinetics, 2002.

Hancock CR, Brault JJ, Terjung RL. Protecting the cellular energy state during contractions: role of AMP deaminase. *J. Physiol. Pharmacol.* 57(Suppl 10):17–29, 2006.

Harris JA Benedict FG A biometric study of human basal metabolism. *Proc Natl Acad Sci U S A.* 4(12): 370–373, 1918 Dec.

Harris JA, Benedict FG. *A Biometric Study of Human Basal Metabolism*. Washington, DC: Carnegie Institution of Washington, 2018.

Harris RC, Stellingwerff T. Effect of β-alanine on high-intensity exercise performance. *Nestle Nutr. Inst. Workshop Ser.* 76:61–71, 2013.

Harris RC, Wise JA, Price KA, Kim HJ, Kim CK, Sale C. Determinants of muscle carnosine content. *Amino Acids* 43:5–12, 2012.

Henneman E. Functional organization of the motorneuron pools. The size principle. In: *Integration of the Nervous System*, pp. 13–25. Eds: Asanuma H, Wilson VJ. Tokyo: Igaku-Shoin, 1979.

Hickson RC Interference of strength development by simultaneously training for strength and endurance. *Eur. J. Appl. Physiol. Occup. Physiol.* 45(2–3):255–263, 1980.

Houmard JA, Scott BK, Justice CL, Chenier TC. The effects of taper on performance in distance runners. *Med. Sci. Sports Exerc.* 26:624–631, 1994.

Horswill CA, Hickner RC, Scott JR, Costill DL, Gould D. Weight loss and dietary carbohydrate modification and high intensity physical performance. *Med. Sci. Sports Exerc.* 22:470–476, 1990.

Hudlicka O. Microcirculation in skeletal muscle. *Muscles Ligaments Tendons J.* 30:3–11, 2011.

Ingjer F. Effects of endurance training on muscle fibre ATP-ase activity, capillary supply and mitochondrial content in man. *J. Appl. Physiol.* 294:419–432, 1979.

Jacobs I, Tesch PA, Bar-Or O, Karlsson J, Dotan R. Lactate in human skeletal muscle after 10 and 30s of supramaximal exercise. *J. Appl. Physiol. Respir. Environ. Exerc. Physiol.* 55:365–367, 1983.

Jacks DE, Sowash J, Anning J, McGloughlin T, Andres F. Effect of exercise at three exercise intensities on salivary cortisol. *J. Strength Cond. Res.* 16:286–289, 2002.

Jansson E, Esbjornsson M, Holm I, Jacobs I. Increase in the proportion of fast-twitch muscle fibres by sprint training in males. *Acta Physiol. Scand.* 140:359–363, 1990.

Jeukendrup AE, Currell K, Clarke J, Cole J, Blannin AK. Effect of beverage glucose and sodium content on fluid delivery. *Nutr. Metab.* 6:9, 2009. doi: 10.1186/1743-7075-6-9.

Karlsson J, Saltin B. Diet, muscle glycogen, and endurance performance. *J. Appl. Physiol.* 31:203–206, 1971.

Kageta T, Tsuchiya Y, Morishima T, Hasegawa Y, Sasaki H, Goto K. Influences of increased training volume on exercise performance, physiological and psychological parameters. *J. Sports Med. Phys. Fitness* 56(7–8):913–921, 2016. Epub 2015 May 15.

Karnincic H, Tocilj Z, Uljevic O, Erceq M. Lactate profile during Greco-Roman wrestling Matchx. *J. Sports Sci. Med.* 8:17–19, 2009.

Katz A, Broberg S, Sahlin K, Wahren,J. Leg glucose uptake during maximal dynamic exercise in humans. *Am. J. Physiol.* 251:E65–E70, 1986.

Kent-Braun JA, McCully KK, Chance B. Metabolic effects of training in humans: a 31P-MRS study. *J. Appl. Physiol.* 69(3):1165–1170, 1990.

Kersick C, Harvey T, Stout J, Campbell B, Wilbom C, Krieder R, Kalman D, Ziegenfuss T, Lopez H, Landin J, Ivy JL, Antonio J. International Society of Sports Nutrition Position Stand: nutrient timing. *J. Int. Soc. of Sports Nutr.* 5:18, 2008.

Kirwan JP, Costill DL, Mitchell JB, Houmard JA, Flynn MG, Fink WJ, Beltz JD. Carbohydrate balance in competitive runners during successive days of intense training. *J. Appl. Physiol.* 65:2601–2606, 1988.

Kley RA, Tarnopolsky MA, Vorgard M. Creatine for treating muscle disorders. *Cochrane Database Syst. Rev.* 5(6):CD004760, 2013.

Knudson DV. Warm-up and flexibility. In: *Conditioning for Strength and Human Performance*, pp. 94–122. Eds: Chandler TJ, Brown LE. Philadelphia, PA: Wolters Kluwer/Lippincott Williams & Wilkins, 2008.

Kraemer WJ, Fleck SJ. *Strength Training for Young Athletes*. Champaign, IL: Human Kinetics, 1993.

Lambert CP. Editorial: is it time for a "muscle-centric" view of maximal oxygen consumption during exercise? *JEP Online* 22(2):1–4, 2019.

Lambert CP, Frank LL, Evans WJ. Macronutrient considerations for the sport of bodybuilding. *Sports Med.* 34:317–327, 2004.

Lambert CP, Jones B. Alternatives to rapid weight loss in U.S. Wrestling. *Int. J. Sports Med.* 31:523–528, 2010.

Lambert CP and Maughan RJ. Influence of beverage temperature on deuterium accumulation in the blood. *Scand. J. Med. Sci. Sports* 2:76–78, 1992.

Lambert CP, Winchester L, Jacks DA, Nader PA. Sex differences in time to fatigue at 100% of VO_2max when normalized for fat free mass. *Res. Sports Med.* 21:78–89, 2013.

Lambert CP. Whole body fat free mass and Vo2peak in recreationally active men and women. *Aerosp. Med. Hum. Perf.* 91:102-105, 2020.

Langfort J, Zarzeczny R, Pilis W, Nazar K, Kaciuba-Uscitko H. The effect of a low carbohydrate diet on performance and metabolic responses to a 30 s bout of supramaximal exercise. *Eur. J. Appl. Physiol.* 76:128–133, 1997.

Layman DK, Evans EM, Erickson D, Seyler J, Weber J, Bagshaw D, Griel A, Psota T, Kris-Etherton P. A moderate protein diet produces sustained weight loss and long term changes in body composition and blood lipids in obese adults. *J. Nutr.* 139:514–521, 2009.

Lemon PW, Dolny DG, Yarasheski KE. Moderate physical activity can increase dietary protein needs. *Can. J. Appl Physiol.* 22:494–503, 1997.

Lemon PW, Tarnopolsky MA, MacDougall JD, Atkinson SA. Protein requirements and muscle mass/strength changes during intensive training in novice bodybuilders. *J. Appl. Physiol.* 73:767–775, 1992.

Litsky F. Wrestling: N.C.A.A plans weight-loss rules. *New York Times*, April 14th Section C, p. 4, 1998. http://www.brianmac.co.uk.

Little JP, Chilibeck PD, Ciona D, Vandenberg A, Zello GA. The effects of low and high glycemic index foods on high intensity intermittent exercise. *Int. J. Sports Phys. Perf.* 4:367–380, 2009.

Magill RA. *Motor Learning: Concepts and Applications*, 2nd Edition. London: W.M. C. Brown Publishers, 1985.

Mah CD, Mah KE, Kezirian EJ, Dement WC. The effect of sleep extension on the athletic performance of collegiate basketball players. *Sleep* 34:943–950, 2011.

Matsui T, Soya M, Soya H. Endurance and brain glycogen: a clue toward understanding central fatigue. *Adv. Neurobiol.* 23:331–346, 2019. doi: 10.1007/978-3-030-27480-1_11.

Maughan RJ, Burke LM, Dvorak KJ, Larson-Meyer DE, Peeling P, Phillips SM, Rawson ES, Walsh NP, Garthe I, Geyer H, Meeusen R. IOC consensus statement dietary supplements and the high performance athlete. *Int. J. Sport Nutr. Excerc. Metab.* 28:104–125, 2018.

Maughan RJ, Gleeson M. Influence of a 36h fast followed by refeeding with glucose, glycerol, or placebo on metabolism during prolonged exercise in man. *Eur. J. Appl. Physiol.* 57:570–576, 1988.

Maughan RJ, Greenhaff PL, Leiper JB, Ball D, Lambert CP, Gleeson M. Diet composition and the performance of high intensity exercise. *J. Sport Sci.* 15:265–275, 1997.

Maughan RJ and Poole DC. The effect of a glycogen loading regimen on the capacity to perform anaerobic exercise. *Eur. J. Appl. Physiol.* 46:211–219, 1981.

McCartney N, Spriet LL, Heigenhauser GJ, Kowalchuck JM, Sutton JR, Jones NL. Maximal power and metabolism in maximal intermittent exercise. *J. Appl. Physiol.* 60:1164–1169, 1986.

McComas AJ. *Skeletal Muscle Form and Function.* Champaign, IL: Human Kinetics, 1996.

McFarlin BK, Flynn MG, Stewart LK, Timmerman KL. Carbohydrate intake during endurance exercise increases natural killer cell responsiveness to IL-2. *J. Appl. Physiol.* 96:271–275, 2004.

McMurray RG, Proctor CR, Wilson WR. Effect of caloric deficit and dietary manipulations on aerobic and anaerobic exercise. *Int. J. Sports Med.* 12:167–172, 1991.

Medbo JI, Mohn AC, Tabata I, Bahr R, Vaage O., Sejerstad OM. Anaerobic capacity determined by maximal accumulated O_2 deficit. *J. Appl. Physiol.* 64:50–60, 1988.

Medbo JI, Tabata I. Anaerobic energy release in working muscle during 30s to 3 min of exhausting bicycling. *J. Appl. Physiol.* 75:1654–1660, 1993.

Melby CL, Schmidt WD, Corrigan D. Resting metabolism rate in weight cycling collegiate wrestlers compared to physically active non-cycling control subjects. *Am. J. Clin. Nutr.* 52:409–414, 1990.

Mettler S, Mitchell N, Tipton KD. Increased protein intake reduces lean body mass loss during weight loss in athletes. *Med. Sci. Sports. Exerc.* 42:326–337, 2010.

Mitchell JB, Costill DL, Houmard JA, Flynn MG, Fink WJ, Beltz JD. Effects of carbohydrate ingestion on gastric emptying and exercise performance. *Med. Sci. Sports Exerc.* 20:110–115, 1988.

Mitchell JB, Costill DL, Houmard JA, Fink WJ, Pascoe DD, Pearson DR. Influence of carbohydrate dosage on exercise performance and glycogen metabolism. *J. Appl. Physiol.* 67:1843–1849, 1989.

Mitchell JB, Phillips MD, Mercer SP, Baylies HL, Pizza FX. Post exercise rehydration: effect of Na^+ and volume on restoration of fluid spaces and cardiovascular function. *J. Appl. Physiol.* 89:1302–1309, 2000.

Montain SJ, Smith SA, Mattot RP, Zientary GP, Jolesz FA, Sawka MN. Hypohydration effects on skeletal muscle performance and metabolism: a 31P-MRS study. *J. Appl. Physiol.* 84:1889–1894, 1998.

Mountjoy ML, Burke LM, Stellingwerff T, Sundgot-Borgen J. Relative energy deficiency in sport: the tip of an iceberg. *Int. J. Sport Nutr. Exerc. Metab.* 28(4):313–315, 2018a. doi: 10.1123/ijsnem.2018-0149. Epub 2018 July 3.

Mountjoy ML, Sundgot-Borgen J, Burke L, Ackerman KE, Blauwet C, Constantini N, Lebrun C, Lundy B, Melin A, Meyer N, Sherman R, Tenforde AS, Torstveit MK, Budgett R. International Olympic Committee (IOC) Consensus Statement on Relative Energy Deficiency in Sport (RED-S): 2018 Update. *Int J Sport Nutr Exerc Metab.* 28(4): 316–331, 2018b. doi: 10.1123/ijsnem.2018-0136. Epub 2018 May 17.

Mujika I. *Tapering and Peaking for Optimal Performance.* Champaign, IL: Human Kinetics, 2009.

Neufer PD, Costill DL, Flynn MG, Kirwan JP, Mitchell JB, Houmard JA. Improvement in exercise performance: effects of carbohydrate feeding and diet. *J. Appl. Physiol.* 62:983–988, 1987.

Nieman DC. Risk of upper respiratory tract infection in athletes: an epidemiologic and immunologic perspective. *J. Athl. Train.* 32:344–349, 1997.

OHSAA Wrestling Weight Certification Assessor Handbook; 2018–2019.

O'Neal EK, Caufield CR, Lowe JB, Stevenson MC, Davis BA, Thigpen L. 24-h fluid kinetics and perception of sweat losses following a 1-h run in a temperate environment. *Nutrients* 6:37–49, 2014.

Parnell JA, Wiens KP, Erdman KA. Dietary intakes and supplement use in pre-adolescent and adolescent Canadian athletes. *Nutrients* 8(9): pii:E526, 2016 August 26. doi: 10.3390/nu8090526.

Poole DC, Burnley M., Vanjatalo A, Rossiter HB, Jones AM. Critical Power: an important fatigue threshold in exercise physiology. *Med Sci Sport Exerc.* 48: 2320–2331, Review, 2016.

Popkin BM, D'Aaci KE, Rosenberg IH. Water, hydration, and health. *Nutrition. Reviews* 68:439–458, 2010.

Padykula J. and Herman E. Factors affecting the activity of adenosine triphosphatase and other phosphatases as measured by histochemical techniques. *Histochem. Cytochem.* 3:161–170, 1955.

Pette D, Ramirez BU, Muller W, Simon R, Exner GU, Hildebrand R. Influence of intermittent long-term stimulation on contractile histochemical and metabolic properties of fibre populations in fast and slow rabbit muscles. *Pflugers Archiv.* 361:1–7, 1975.

Reid MB. Redox interventions to increase exercise performance. *J. Physiol.* 594(18):5125–5133, 2016. doi: 10.1113/JP270653. Epub 2015 December 20.

Roemmich JN, Sinning WE. Weight loss and wrestling training effects on nutrition, growth, maturation, body composition, and strength. *J. Appl. Physiol.* 82:1751–1759, 1987a.

Roemmich JN, Sinning WE. Weight loss and wrestling training effects on growth related hormones. *J. Appl. Physiol.* 82:1760–1764, 1987b.

Ross LM, Barber JL, McLain AC, Weaver RG, Sui X, Blair SN, Sarzynski MA. The association of cardiorespiratory fitness and ideal cardiovascular health in the aerobics center longitudinal study. *J. Phys. Act Health.* 24:1–8, 2019. doi: 10.1123/jpah.2018-0220.

Ross R, Blair, SN, Arena R, Church TS, Despres JP, Franklin BA, Haskell WL, Kaminsky LA, Levine BD, Lavie CJ, Myers J, on behalf of the American Heart Association Physical Activity Committee of the Council on Lifestyle and Cardiometabolic Health, Council on Clinical Cardiology, Council on Epidemiology and Prevention, Council on Cardiovascular and Stroke Nursing, Council on Genomic and Precision Medicine; and Stroke Council. Importance of assessing cardiorespiratory fitness in clinical practice: a case for fitness as a clinical vital sign: a scientific statement from the American Heart Association. *Circulation* 134:00–00, 2016. doi: 10.1161/CIR.0000000000000461.

Rushall BS. A tool for measuring stress tolerance in elite athletes. *J. Appl. Sport Psych.* 2:51–66, 1990.

Sale DG. Neural adaptations to resistance training. *Med. Sci. Sports Exerc.* 20(5 Suppl):S135–S145, 1988.

Saltin B. Aerobic and anaerobic work capacity after dehydration. *J. Appl. Physiol.* 19:1114–1118, 1964.

Sawka MN, Burke LM, Eichner ER, Maughan RJ, Montain SJ, Stachenfeld NS. ACSM Position Stand. Exercise and fluid replacement. *Med. Sci Sports Exerc.* 39:377–390, 2007.

Schmidt WD, Corrigan D, Melby CL. Two seasons of weight cycling does not lower resting metabolic rate in college wrestlers. *Med. Sci. Sports Exerc.* 25:613–619, 1993.

Sharp RL. Role of sodium in fluid homeostasis with exercise. *J. Am. Coll. Nutr.* 25:231S–239S, 2006.

Shepley B, MacDougall JD, Cipriano N, Sutton JR, Tarnopolsky MA, Coates G. Physiological effects of tapering in highly trained athletes. *J. Appl. Physiol.* 72:706–711, 1992.

Sherman WM, Costill DL, Fink WJ, Miller JM. Effects of exercise-diet manipulation on muscle glycogen and its subsequent utilization during performance. *Int. J. Sports Med.* 2:1–15, 1981.

Sherman WM, Peden MC, Wright DA. Carbohydrate feeding 1 h before exercise improve cycling performance. *Am. J. Clin. Nutr.* 54:866–870, 1991.

Shoemaker JK, Green HJ, Ball-Burnett M, Grant S. Relationships between fluid and electrolyte hormones and plasma volume during exercise with training and detraining. *Med. Sci. Sports Exerc.* 30(4):497–505, 1998.

Simonson JC, Sherman WM, Lamb DR, Dernbach AR, Doyle JA, Strauss R. Dietary carbohydrate, muscle glycogen, and power output during rowing training. *J. Appl. Physiol.* 70:1500–1505, 1991.

Snyder AC, Kuipers H, Cheng B, Servais R, Fransen E. Overtraining following intensified training with normal muscle glycogen. *Med. Sci. Sports Exerc.* 27:1063–1070, 1995.

Spencer MK, Katz A. Role of glycogen in control of glycolysis and IMP formation in human muscle during exercise. *Am. J. Physiol.* 260:E859–E864, 1991.

Spina RJ, Chi MM, Hopkins MG, Nemeth PM, Lowry OH, Holloszy JO. Mitochondrial enzymes increase in muscle in response to 7–10 days of cycle exercise. *J. Appl. Physiol.* 80:2250–2254, 1996.

Spriet LL. Exercise and sport performance with low dose caffeine. *Sports Med.* 44(Suppl 2):S175–S184, 2014.

Stellingwerf T, Maughan RJ, Burke LM. Nutrition for power sports, middle distance running, rack cycling, rowing, canonoing/kayaking, and swimming. *J. Sports Sci.* 29:579–589, 2011.

Stellingwerf T, Spriet L, Watt M, Kinder N, Hargreaves M, Hawley J, Burky, LM. Decreased PDH activation and glycogenolysis during exercise following fat adaptation with carbohydrate restoration. *Am. J. Physiol. Endo. Metab.* 290:E380–E388, 2006.

Stone MH, Stone ME. Strength and conditioning for sport. In: *Conditioning for Strength and Human Performance*, pp. 94–122. Eds: Chandler TJ, Brown LE. Philadelphia, PA: Wolters Kluwer/Lippincott Williams & Wilkins, 2008.

Stryer L. *Biochemistry*, 3rd Edition. New York, NY: W.H. Freeman and Company, 1988.

Tabata I, Nishimura K, Kovzaki M, Hirai Y, Ogita F, Miyachi M, Yamamoto K. Effects of moderate-intensity endurance and high-intensity intermittent training on anaerobic capacity and VO_2max. *Med. Sci. Sports Exerc.* 28:1327–1330, 1996.

Tallon MJ, Harris RC, Boobis LH, Fallowfield JL, Wise JA. The carnosine content of vastus lateralis is elevated in resistance-trained bodybuilders. *J. Strength Cond. Res.* 19:725–729, 2005.

Tesch PA, Thorsson A, Essen-Gustavsson B. Enzyme activities of FT and ST muscle fibers in heavy resistance trained individuals. *J. Appl. Physiol.* 67:83–87, 1989.

Tipton KD, Elliott TA, Cree MC, Wolf SE, Sanford AP, Wolfe RR. Ingestion of casein and whey proteins result in muscle anabolism after resistance exercise. *Med. Sci. Sports Exerc.* 36:2075–2081, 2004.

Trappe S, Costill D, Thomas R. Effect of a swim taper on whole muscle and single muscle fiber contractile properties. *Med. Sci. Sports Exerc.* 33:48–56, 2000.

Trappe S, Luden N, Minchev K, Raue U, Jemiolo B, Trappe TA. Skeletal muscle signature of a champion sprint runner. *J. Appl. Physiol.* 118:1460–1466, 2015.

Trappe S, Williamson D, Godard M. Maintenance of whole muscle strength and size following resistance training in older men. *J. Gerontol. A. Biol. Sci. Med. Sci.* 57:B138–B143, 2002.

Trappe TA. Titin and nebulin content in human skeletal muscle following eccentric resistance exercise. *Muscle & Nerve* 25:289–292, 2002.

Trexler ET, Smith-Ryan AE, Stout JR, Hoffman JR, Wilborn CD, Sale C, Kreider RB, Jäger R, Earnest CP, Bannock L, Campbell B, Kalman D, Ziegenfuss TN, Antonio J. International Society of Sports Nutrition Position Stand: beta-alanine. *J. Int. Soc. Sports Nutr.* 12:30, 2015. doi: 10.1186/s12970-015-0090-y.

USA Wrestling Coach's Guide to Excellence, 2nd Edition. Traverse City, MI: Cooper Publishing Group, LLC, 2005.

Watson G, Judelman DA, Armstrong LE, Yeargin SW, Casa DJ, Maresh CM. Influence of diuretic induced dehydration on competitive sprint and power performance. *Med. Sci. Sports Exerc.* 37:1168–1174, 2005.

Westererp KR. Diet induced thermogenesis. *Nutr. Metab.* 1:1–5, 2004.

Wilmore JH, Costill DL. *Physiology of Sport and Exercise.* Champaign, IL: Human Kinetics, 1994.

Yang J, Christophi CA, Fariola A, Baur DM, Moffatt S, Zollinger TW, Kales SN. Association between push-up exercise capacity and future cardiovascular events among active adult men. *JAMA Netw. Open.* 2(2):e188341, 2019. doi: 10.1001/jamanetworkopen.2018.8341.

Index

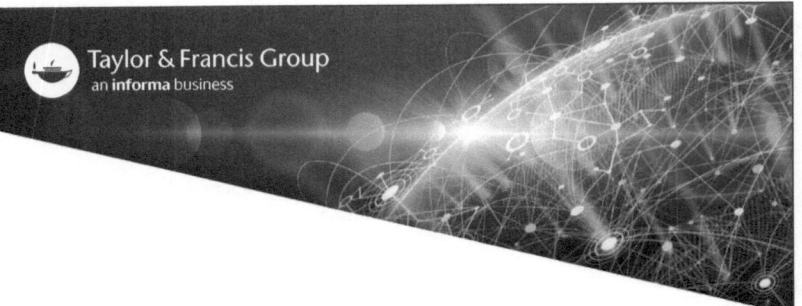
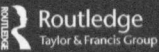
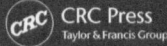